Passion Profession & Politics

Autobiography of the American Chiropractor

Who Became Chief Physician of the Olympic Team of the *USSR*

Dr. Stephen J. Press

NB - All case histories, when mentioning actual names, are by written permission of the patient. Some names have been changed to hide the identities of certain individuals.

ISBN 0-7414-2213-1

Published by:

INFINITY
PUBLISHING.COM

1094 New DeHaven Street, Suite 100
West Conshohocken, PA 19428-2713
Info@buybooksontheweb.com
www.buybooksontheweb.com
Toll-free (877) BUY BOOK
Local Phone (610) 941-9999
Fax (610) 941-9959

Printed in the United States of America

Printed on Recycled Paper

Published February 2005

Passion
Profession
& Politics

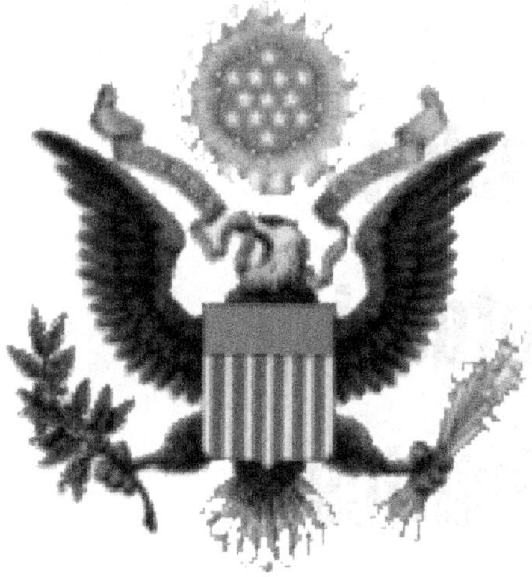

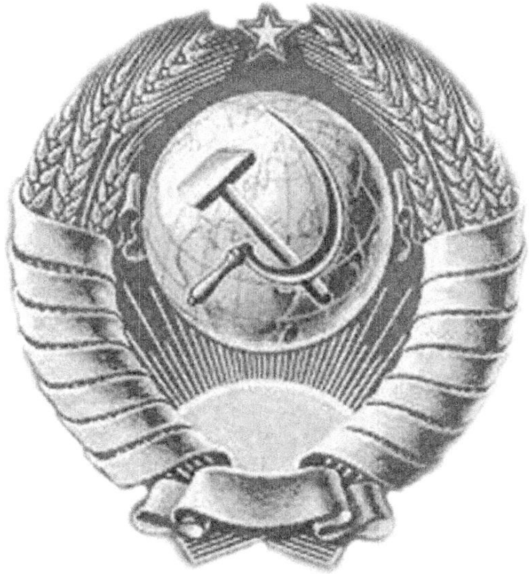

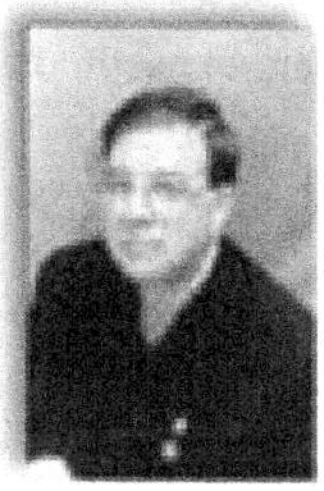

Dr. Stephen Jay Press

Brief Professional Biography

BA, Biological Sciences, Thomas Edison College, NJ
DC - Doctor of Chiropractic, Palmer College, 1978
Board Certified Chiro. Sports Physician, National College, 1980
Fellow, American College of Sports Medicine, 1983
(World's only DC to hold this title)

Diplomate, Fédération Int'le de la Mèdicine du Sports, Course, 1986
Fellow, International College of Chiropractors, ca 1993
PhD (Cand.), Intercontinental University, Ltd., Moscow, Russia

Staff Doctor, Preakness Hospital, Wayne, N.J. – Passaic County Facility
Staff Privileges, Fort Lee Surgical Center
Manipulation under Anesthesia

Board Member, American Chiropractic Assoc. Sports Council, 1986-87
Chairman, International Affairs Committee
Chairman, 1987 PanAm Games,
Chiro. Speaker selection committee

Medical Director, Jersey Shore Marathon ca, 1985, 86
Medical Director, World Arm Wrestling Championships,
England, ca 1987

Founder, Fédération Internationale de Chiropratique du Sports, 1987
Pres., Fédération Internationale de Chiropratique du Sports, 1987-1991
Recipient, FICS Gold Medal, Life honorary member 1991

Listed, "*America's Best Chiropractors*" 2004
Listed, International Who's Who in Medicine

US National Team Doctor, World Tae Kwon Do Championships,
Madison Sq. Garden, NYC, 1993
Chief Physician, Winter Olympic Team of the Soviet Union 1992
XVIth Winter Olympic Games, Albertville, France

Pres, Medical Comm., Féd. Internationale de Roller Sports 1998-2000
Vice-Pres., Medical Comm., Féd. Internationale des Échecs 2000-2003

Founder & Chairman,
Int'l Academy of Olympic Chiropractic Officers 1978
Founder, President, Russian Chiropractic Association, 1990- Present
Founder, Chairman, Eastern European Chiropractic Union, 1990-Present

TABLE of CONTENTS

FOREWORD

Dr. Stephen Press, born in the Bronx, grew up to become a Doctor of Chiropractic, rose to become Founder and then Chairman of the World Governing Body for his professional specialty, got appointed Chief Physician of the Olympic Team of the Soviet Union and Presided over the formation of not one but two Medical Commissions of IOC (International Olympic Committee) recognized International Sports Federations.

He was the personal Doctor for many world and Olympic names, especially in figure skating, and traveled all over the planet, teaching, and treating Athletes and ordinary folk alike.

This book, an introspective autobiography, takes a look back at the "*Concussion of Forces*" and serendipitous events that shaped his sometimes rocky personal and economic life, the tragedy of an unfulfilled love affair, and the developments that shaped and guided his extraordinary professional career. He shares many behind-the-scenes stories about the many celebrities he has known and treated, and the history he participated in molding.

TABLE of FIGURES

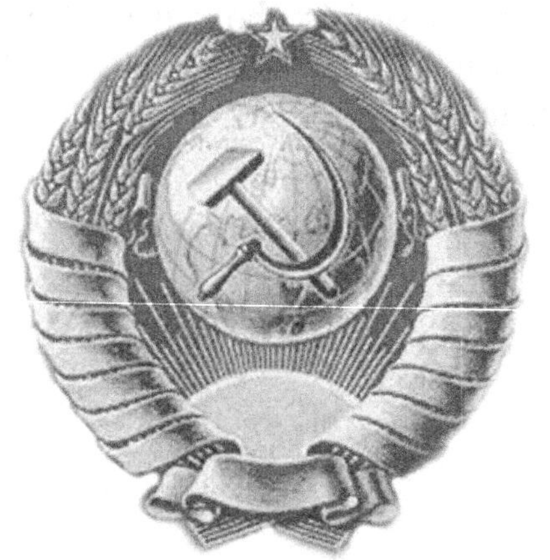

PROLOGUE

I have been privileged to have lived a life filled with excitement. I've been to many, many interesting places, and seen many unique things. Professionally, I started out to be the best Sports Chiropractor I could be. Money was always of secondary importance to me, and always was seen as merely a means towards the end of accomplishing what I set out to do.

It was serendipity that put me in the place I found myself, and serendipity that brought me to the place I attained. Naturally there were always others on whom I had to rely for help and those who were voluntarily there to give my life direction, and I could have accomplished none of what I did without their help, for which I shall always be grateful.

Starting at an early age, there were many times in my life that I was despised, or was the subject of jealous distrust from those around me. I guess it was that experience and resultant qualities which allowed me to shrug off the weight of starting a World agency. Dr. Ron Harris, a former Officer of the ACA once told me; "*every time you take a step up... someone will be aiming at you*". You have to be able to handle that.

Probably, had I been always happy at home, I would not have felt the need to bury myself in my profession, and perhaps a lot of the professional accomplishments would not have occurred. In retrospect, I would gladly have traded the one for the other.

After being the only American named "*Chief Physician*" for the Soviet Olympic Team, and being in the right place at the right time to become Founder of the World Governing Body for the professional specialty of Sports Chiropractic, one does ask "*where to now*"? How do I top that? I did.... As to what more I can accomplish, only the future will tell... I'll just keep on being me.... What you see is what you get.

Dedication

I want to thank all the many people who have been there when I needed them. Some were later were to take advantage of their position, some even turned on me as soon as they had a chance to so, but even they were there at some point, and for the constructive things they contributed, I thank all of them. Those who were always there, and were always my friends, I want thank especially…..from the depths of my heart.

I want to dedicate this book to my parents, and to my Sons, Robert and Yuri, and finally but not at all least, to my beloved Olga, who, though she came only recently into my life, has so changed it for the better, that I shall never be the same person.

Thanks

Many thanks to Tom Hyde, DC; Gordon Lawson, DC; Bill Cirino, Sr., DC; and Saul Liss, PhD, and H.E., Count Robert Maurice Von Glück und Kuefstein, for all of your support, and friendship through times good and bad. To Professor Clint Strong of IU, Vojin Smodlaka, MD, and Allan Ryan, MD, to Prof. Aleshinsky, Sergei Yurievich to Minister Rusak, Anatoly Ivanovich, and Prof. Dr. Popov, Sergie Nikolaievich. And last but not least to Sr. Isidro Oliveras of Barcelona who believed in me, supported me, and gave a Chiropractor a chance at something no Chiropractor had ever done before.

Chapter I

Lineage and Beginnings

**

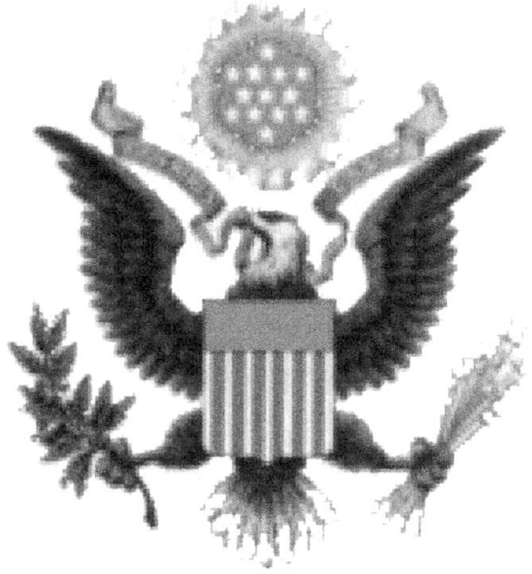

Though Jews don't believe in Hell, they must have experienced it being Jewish in Middle Ages Europe. It was in 1450 that this family starts tracing its roots, when Simon Sacke the Younger left Konstanz, Prussia near Switzerland with his wife Gütlin, to make what was then a long trek to Frankfort. They couldn't own property, had no civil rights, and were forced into certain jobs that only Jews were allowed to hold. Before long the Jewish sector of Frankfort would be leveled by the secular authorities, and the entire Jewish community would be evicted en masse. Forced out of town, they founded a new ghetto at what is now called Offenbach am main, not far from the center of Frankfort.

The Ox' feet

Simon built a home for his family, and, in the tradition of the time, put a sort of coat of arms on the door, the foot of an ox was the illustration he chose, for reasons unknown today, and thus his home was called Rindsfüss, (ox's foot). Families came to be known by their signs, and they were called the Rindsfüsses. After a couple of generations, one of their descendants decided that an Ox' head was more propitious then the feet, and upgraded the family crest, when he enlarged the living quarters, calling the renovated home Rindskopf (ox's head). Thus the family was known for some three centuries in those parts. They became highly prominent in banking, and grew to a stature on the order of and at times exceeding the Rothschild family. Prospering until one day some Baron borrowed an enormous sum to finance a war, and failing to repay, nearly bankrupted the Rindskopf fortune.

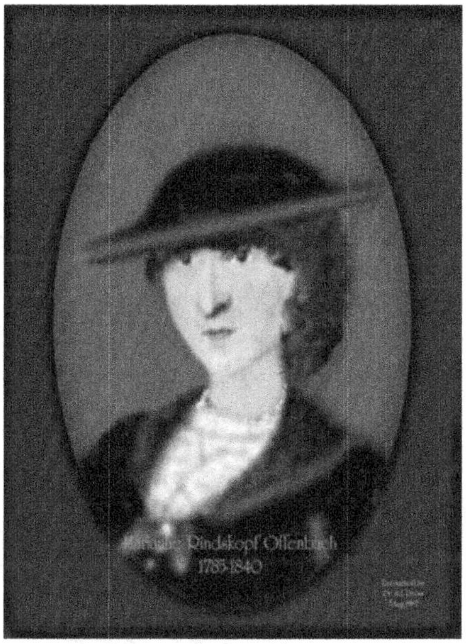

Fig 1 Marianne Rindskopf Offenbach
The author's 4th great Grandmother

Around the end of the 18th Century, Marianne Rindskopf, married Isaac, whose family's marking/name is now believed, according to [1]Jacobo Kaufmann's book, to have been "*Eberstadt*", and the newlyweds started having children, at the then reasonable rate of one every two years. Around 1810, Marianne and Isaac moved to Köln, and Isaac, who had been a tutor to the Rothschilds, found work as cantor at the great synagogue there, where his statue still graces the town square.

---

[1] Isaac Offenbach und sein sohn Jacques oder "*Es is nicht alle Tage Purim*", Jacobo Kaufmann, 1998, Max Niemeyer Verlag, Tübingen, Germany

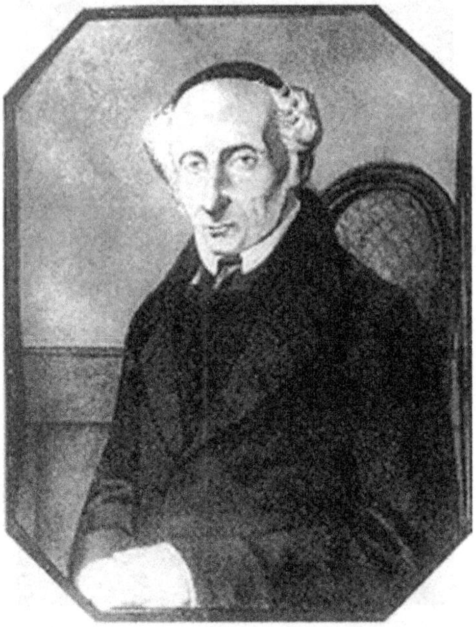

Fig 2 Isaac Eberstadt Offenbach
The author's 4th great Grandfather

In Köln, he was soon known as Isaac der Offenbacher. So, when Napoleon's edict came to roost in 1817, that all Jews must take inheritable family names, it was a short jump to becoming [2]Isaac Offenbach. Among his ultimately nine offspring, were Jacob and Jules. All the children were musical, and at an early age Jacob and his brother were trod off to far away Paris for what Dad considered a real musical education. It was only in Paris that Jacob became known as "*Jacques*", and the rest of his story, is shall we say history.

It bears note there, that it would appear that I am not the only member of this enormous extended family to gravitate

[2] The author has a copy of Jacque's birth certificate, showing that at this time his father was already known as Isaac Offenbach.

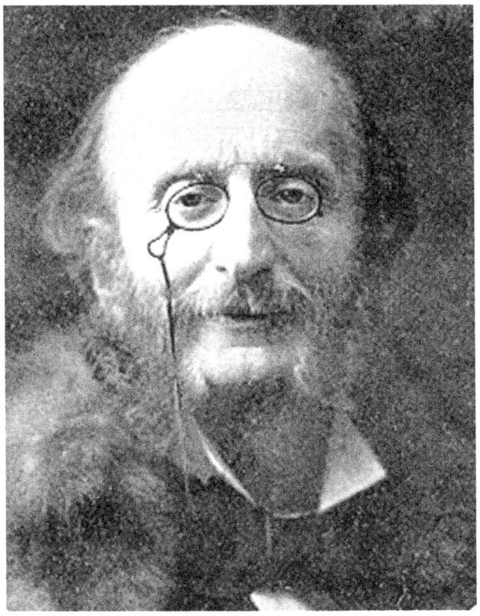

Fig 3 Jacob Jacques Offenbach
The Author's 3rd great Uncle

towards International sport. I am informed by my 6th cousin, Yves Brindejont-Offenbach , that Pierre Comte-Offenbach, a 5th Cousin once removed, was a member of the IOC, from France.

A Great Composer

Several of Jacques' sisters married rather successfully, and at least three finally came to America, founding their own family dynasties; the Maas' of Southern department store chain fame; the Grüenewalds/McCorkles, founders of the Delaware-Maryland-Virginia telephone company, and others. One sister, exactly which one we are not certain, sent her offspring here to avoid the by then compulsory military service which the Prussian government in granting Jews civil rights, mandated. It was especially urgent because they were in the middle of the Franco-Prussian war, and with Jacques and Jules being already rather well known and having adopted French citizenship, any family left in Cologne would have been seen as possible collaborators.

Rebecca and Israel came here through England, we think, and took the name Silbermann, which got anglicized to Silverman pretty quickly. Whether Rebecca and Israel were themselves the Sister and Brother-in-Law, or Brother and Sister-in-law of the Composer, or his Niece or Nephew, we are not yet certain. What we do have is a strong family tradition that Offenbach was the Uncle of my Great Grandma Sarah (Rebecca's daughter), and we have all heard down the line, that this was a name taken from papers bought from a dead Polish soldier who obviously no longer needed them. Though there is still a mystery about why they would have needed a false identity? Almost anyone was welcomed here at that time; around 1870, and we can't imagine why they would have needed phony papers to get out of Prussia.... unless perhaps to avoid what was then a twenty year military service obligation for their son. Although, why not then on arrival, proclaim your true identity, and reassume your famous name?

In any event it comes as no surprise then, that the several offspring of Rebecca and Israel, on gaining majority changed their own names to variations on Silverman. The Silvern's married into the Gladstones who also came through a sojourn in England, and the Gladstones begat Isabella, who married Sam Graf, and they begat Rénee, whose union with Howard Press brought me into the line.

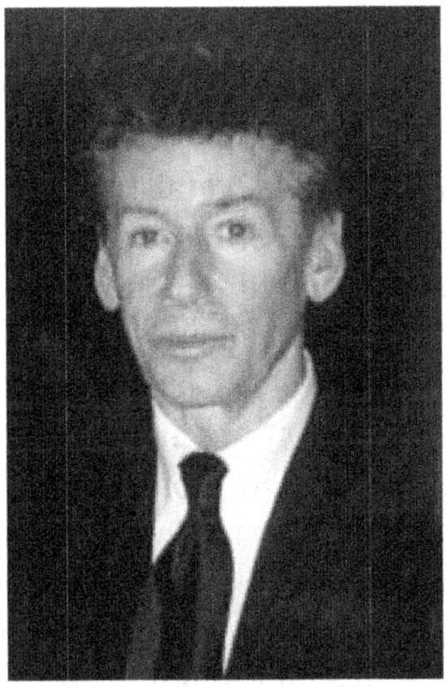

Fig 4 Calvin Klein
the Author's 2nd Cousin

CK

On my mom's father's side, were the Graf's, a family of furriers, who came here around the turn of the 20th century, ostensibly to avoid anti-semitism in the Carpathian alps region, on the Romanian side of the border, in a little town named Culcurea Mare (great cross), near Chernowitz, in what is now Ukraine. From that couple, whose nine children alone have on last count given me some 454 relatives, also included several notables. Sam's sister Molka (Molly) married one of the only shady characters I found; a dentist who, rumor has it, ran off to join up with Al Capone in the 20's leaving Molly and their daughter Flore, practically destitute. Flore would later marry Leo Klein and their child Calvin of clothing design fame, is thereby my second cousin.

Another member of the Graf line, married Samuel Bronner, the man who built the Plaza Hotel, and another Mildred Geller, married Himan Brown, the man who produced the famous radio show "*the Shadow*".

I actually didn't know that the great Calvin was my cousin until just a few years ago, when my genealogical interests took me to a new look at the Graf line. When I started making calls, I was asked several times by members of the family, if I had "*spoken to Calvin yet?*" I incredulously took his mom's phone number to call her, only to find that the first time I called was the evening they took his dad Leo to the hospital on the eve of his passing. It was to be some months before I called back, as it was rather uncomfortable to bring back the memory to Flore of our first conversation, and I just didn't know how to begin. However, when I did finally call her again, she was most gracious about it, and after losing herself a bit in her praising of her son's status as a member of the family and how generous and what a good son he was, etc., she gave me the names, dates, and places I needed from her. She also promised to mention me to Calvin, and a few weeks later after I sent him a preliminary chart of my work to that point, he called my office.

My secretary at that time, who was accustomed to receiving calls from other celebrities in sports, went completely bonkers over talking to Calvin.

We discussed the idea of a family reunion one day, and when I sent him the completed chart in time for his mom's 90th birthday party, he called again. This time it was to invite me and Tanya to the party. What he left out was that he had arranged to send the corporate jet all over the US picking up cousins he found out about in my chart; put them all up in suites at the incredible hotel Pierre, and set up hot and cold running Mercedes S class limos to take everyone around town during their stay.

The party was at le Cirque, and to say the least, it left a lasting impression on everyone who was invited.

The best things for me were really twofold; one, that my mom got re-united with a long lost set of her first cousins, some of whom had moved to within nearly walking distance of her in Florida and with whom she is now once again close; and two, that he had his in-house advertising firm arrange to print my chart as a book, in full color and bound to pass out to the family attending the party! Class.

Polliwitz

Dad's side was not so filled with famous folk. His people came from what is now the capital of Lithuania, today called Vilnius, and also from the Capital of what is now Belarus, in Minsk. Their offspring produced a host of medical professionals and a few lawyers. The name Press, it seems wasn't always Press. In Belarus, my paternal forebears were known by something akin to Polavetz, then anglicizing it to Pollowitz. Press is also a known Jewish family name there, especially in the region around Gomel, and I suspect from hints in the documents and from things related by elders, that Jacob Pollowitz's wife's maiden name was Press, and they just changed it like so many did to Americanize the name and, by using her family name, kept one of their family lines' names alive.

At least I didn't find any horse-thieves or murderers.

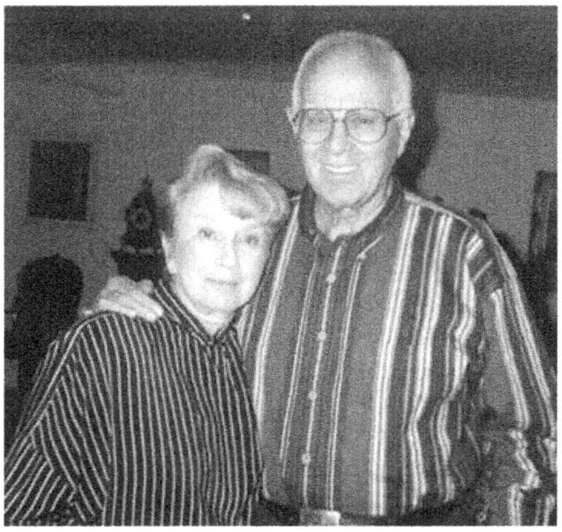

Fig 5 The Author's parents, Howard and Renee

Holland Ave.

Cedars of Lebanon Hospital – Bronx, NY – "*Baby boy*" Press is born to Renée and Howard Press. Next day he's given the name Stephen Jay. They thought about Xavier, but that would have made me X Press, and Stephen Allen, but they didn't like those initials.

We were living in a one bedroom apartment at 2141 Holland Ave., in the Bronx, which we shared with my maternal Grandmother, Bella, née Isabella Gladstone. It was near the corner of Lydig Ave. It was a Jewish "*shtetl*". A virtually 100% Jewish area. In fact it would be only in PS 105 that I would discover what a Christian was... i.e., only the faculty were non Jews. In retrospect, it seems pretty funny how we went to "*auditorium*" at holidays, and were taught Christmas carols.... A school composed virtually 100% of Jewish kids proficiently singing Adeste Fideles in Latin!

Mom is a unique blend of Eastern and Western European Jewry, though we were never the ones for real religion. She recalls being teased as the only Jewish girl in her class, whose "*Bubba*" (Grandmother) didn't keep Kosher. No dummy my mom, she graduated from Hunter College at 19, where she majored in Biology and minored in French.

Dad was a pharmacy student before the War, and because of his education, lucked out in the European theatre, where he was assigned to a hospital as a lab technician, doing urine and fecal analyses. But at least he was able to continue his education in Europe. So, he studied in England and then after the liberation of Paris, at the famous Sorbonne.

My folks were doting parents, taking me to see Bill Baird's marionette shows, the circus, and to museums, and even children's opera... the Love of Three Oranges was a highlight. We went on trips to Cape Cod (till there was a

Polio scare) and then to Miami. I had them to myself until Richard Heath came along at age nine.

Rich Appears

Then my life changed completely. This little "*angel*", with his blonde curls and his way of making everyone adore him, was in many ways my antithesis. And, I suppose like my classmates, he too, took perverse delight in tormenting me from a very early age. Being nine years his senior left me the one to baby-sit whenever mom and dad went out. And, since I was the elder sibling, I took full responsibility for whatever went wrong, whether it was something I had control over or not.

From age seven I began to play with chemistry, and had a rather extensive "*chemistry set*", far exceeding the chemicals specifically juxtaposed in the commercially available toy sets, due to reasons we'll discuss later. This meant that there were really poisonous substances in my care. I was old enough not to put them in my mouth, and when Richard began to walk, I asked to leave my room locked when I was out. Request denied, subject closed! Reason? I was told that this was only due to sibling jealousy and that I just didn't want him playing with my things. In reality I adored my brother, and was really just trying to protect him from a possibly serious accident.

One day I came home from school, and found "*pretty*" blue crystals on the floor in the center of my room. I freaked, as this was copper sulfate, which is really toxic, and I knew that it had to have been Rich who was a toddler and had obviously been playing in my chemicals. Again, mom took it as a jealousy thing, and basically ignored my pleas to check him out. Thanks God he never actually put anything in his mouth.... Maybe the Press' were just born to play with chemicals?

Prow and Dad's Businesses

The era of my birth makes me a "*baby boomer*". Mom and dad married before he left for Europe. When he got back, he went into business with my Grandma Bella's Brother-in-Law, my great uncle, Lou Morrow, and together they formed Prow Chemical Co., which made them a pretty good income for several years afterwards. Prow was a brokerage, which found stores of needed chemicals and put them together with needy buyers. One year, about 1953 I suppose, they grossed more than a million dollars in sales.

But Lou got greedy, and decided that they could expand by buying up inventory. Dad told me he felt this was the kiss of death in that business where every need was so ephemeral. And they disbanded the firm.

Time Release

Later he got into pharmaceutical manufacturing, making pills for doctors who had their own private formulae, and eventually got the idea to create a form of nitroglycerine that could dissolve over time. He was awarded the first process patent for the concept of "*time release*". We should have been billionaires from that alone. But he lost a 17 year war with the biggest companies in the world, who just decided that theft would get them what they wanted. Later, he would pay a very severe price for fighting for what he believed in.

I can recall like yesterday, standing at my mother's knee at the secretary desk that I now have in my bedroom; begging her to teach me to read. I must have been four. But Dr. Spock's was the child-rearing bible of the day, and he said that it would leave me bored in class when other kids were first learning to read, so I had to wait. Then I got to kindergarten, and Sherry Barrack could read, and I was so jealous, so I tried again, but to no avail. Dr. Spock won the day.

It was a similar battle when I started first grade. Mom regaled me with stories about how she had graduated at 19, but her cousin Missie had graduated Hunter at only 18. I recall how I set a goal to compete with their records. They could skip grades, because the school allowed for a 1A, 1B system. I recall my utter horror when on the first day of class, I was told that the School system had just eliminated skipping. I was devastated.... Still remember thinking "*oh my God! I'm condemned to spending six whole years here?*" At that, I lost my desire to do well in school, for a very long time.

There must have been something besides this trauma in 1st grade that keeps me from remembering the face of Mrs. Groveman. Was she abusive? What could it have been about her? I could work with a Police sketch artist to draw the faces of all my grammar school teachers even today.... Except her. Only Mrs. Groveman I cannot recall at all.

About this time, someone gave me a record, called "*Rusty in Orchestraville*". It was a charming story about a child who falls asleep playing scales on the piano. He hates playing his scales, and curses the piano. In his dream, he meets the Conductor of Orchestraville, who introduces him one by one to all the instruments, who are now sentient beings. As Rusty befriends them, they allow him to play them and he can magically play the most beautiful or difficult piece ever written for that instrument. Naturally the piano doesn't want to talk to him, because of the nasty things he said about it while falling asleep. But eventually even the piano allows him to play it, and he plays the minute waltz by Hayden. During the course of the story he plays the cello, and I am entranced by the sound of the Swan by Saint Saen.

The Cello

After that, I wanted only to play the cello. So, mom took me to the Fordham Academy of Music, where I was asked what

I wanted to do. Naturally I wanted the cello, and only the cello. But we were convinced that it would be really hard to get a small cello for such a little boy to play, so perhaps I should take a music appreciation course for a year, and then decide.

At the end of my year, I still would hear only of the cello, so we were introduced to a cousin of Rob Reiner's, Sam, who was teaching there part-time, but unknown to us at the time was a well known Broadway show cellist. Mr. Reiner agreed to come to the apartment to teach me privately. We didn't know his reason for accepting me at the time, but later he would tell my mother that he had thought I might be related to the great Joseph Press, a famous cellist, of whom we had never heard.

Mom told him innocently enough that we were no relations of Joseph Press', and the only musician in our family was the composer Offenbach. It was Reiner who told her that Offenbach was a cellist. This connection was to start me later on another hobby, genealogy.

Languages

When I was little, due to dad's French education, and mom's college French, they spoke French at home so I wouldn't understand. Children though absorb languages like sponges, so after I started to catch on, they switched to the smattering of German they both had been forced to study in college.

Later, I was forced to study Hebrew to prepare for Bar Mitzvah, and though I really never learned Hebrew, this, plus a Sixth grade teacher, Mrs. Cinelli, who spoke seven languages fluently, really influenced my linguistic future.

In school, since I was so bored, reading at 12th grade level in 3rd grade, I simply lost interest, and frequently flunked classes due to failure to participate or turn in homework assignments. In retrospect, I must have frustrated my teachers and parents half to death.

I will never forget a confrontation in 3rd grade with Mrs. Patrick, who really did care about me. I showed up one morning without a now overdue book report. So she demanded "*where was the report*?" I told her I had forgotten to do it, but had read the book. So she made me sit at the rear of the room and just go write the report. Naturally, I hadn't read the requisite book either. So I just made one up whole cloth. The Author too! My report on "*The Icy Continent*", about Antarctica, was a hit, I got an "A".

Illness strikes

At about age 8, I started to notice that I had blood in my urine. And my mom, being a trained biologist at least knew this was something to run, not walk to the pediatrician with. Dr. Harry Seif, was in the flat-iron building near Fordham Rd. He ran some tests and then, more from intuition than science, ordered me to bed-rest, and on antibiotics, which were still rather a new thing in those days. I stayed home and virtually bed-ridden for three months! Grandma Bella was at my side almost every day, and my mom, who was pregnant with what would have been her second child, was carrying me around and dragging things she probably should not have been, but had to because of my illness. She lost a baby some years earlier, and hinted that she risked losing my brother through caring for me at home. I was diagnosed as having "acute glomerulo-nephritis" by Dr. Seif, who likely saved my life, as those who become chronic rarely make it past 35.

Tormented in School

In grade school, I talked a good line, but when the kids found out I got lousy grades, and for whatever other personality reasons, they generally hated me. Frequently I was followed home by bands of hooligans shouting anti-gay epithets and challenging my manhood. I always knew my own sexuality was not an issue, and would have none of their garbage, thus further fueling their rage. This was clearly an era in which, had I beaten up a brat or two, the torment would have stopped. But, I stubbornly refused to lower myself to their level. As a result, school became a living Hell for me, made all the worse by my penchant for staying up late, and being unable to function in the wee hours of the morning, like 8:00AM.

Having screwed myself with lousy grades, I was not considered for Bronx Science, where I certainly would have been at home. That to be truthful, was hard to take. But, I really did bring it on myself. Despite the lack of this recognition for my intellect, I was the quintessential science nerd, except for the all important grade thing. When the other kids were playing ball, I was in my lab at home, doing chemical experiments.

Since Dad was in the pharmaceutical manufacturing business, and had a lab at work; Grandma Bella worked at Clay Adams, a surgical supply place; my Cousin Jack was a Chemistry professor at City College; and even my Dad's partner's son was studying Chemistry at Fordham, I had a constant influx of supplies, chemicals, glassware etc. So, by the time I got to College, I could do organic analysis at home more efficiently than in the University Lab at Fairleigh Dickinson.

So, after Grammar School, I was forced to go to the "*lower class*" Jr. High, PS 83, and endured that environment, where in some ways it was even worse than at 105 for a half year. Finally, thankfully, my folks found a house in then all WASP Tenafly. We were the first or second family of Jewish background to move to Tenafly, and I caught it in school for that.

In Tenafly Jr. High School, I immediately gravitated toward the other nerdy guys, and made all the wrong friends. Harrison Pierce Reed, III, was uniformly despised in class, and we became immediate buddies.

Here, I continued my attitude about homework, and kept getting lousy grades, despite that I was really learning everything I was taught. Borrrring! And Gym... well I quickly found out that this was where the bullies could "*get*" the guys they didn't like. There was little to no supervision in the locker rooms, and I was always picked on there. Thus I developed medical excuses to keep me from taking much Gym. And, it helped that I suffered from serious allergic attacks. This just compounded the problem, so I retreated into extracurricular activities like Library, and Stage Crew, and other nerdy things that only served to make the class think I was less manly than the jocks. I got teased again and again about my masculinity. Always that.... Why did they think I was Gay? Strange....

Maybe today that's why I am so sensitive to the plight of gay men and lesbians. Imagine the Hell I went through when kids just called me that to torment me, suppose I had actually been gay? My God!

Anti-Semitism

When I got to Tenafly Jr. High, where I was probably the first Jewish kid there, it was not without repercussions. I took Anti-Semitic jokes from the other kids. But I did not expect to have to cope with that from the faculty too.

The Music plot

Since I was the new kid on the block and was a bit traumatized at the transition anyway, I didn't enroll immediately in the school orchestra, despite having played cello in PS 105 for the prior 5 years. So, Mr. X, the music appreciation teacher, also was not aware of my musical background, and thus, I guess he thought he could "*get the Jewish kid*", or whatever sick reasons he had to hurt me scholastically.

Whenever I turned in homework I got zeros! In Music appreciation! I knew that I had answered the questions correctly, but still got zeros! Tests too... all zeros! What to do?

Luckily, though I didn't know it, a really nice guy was living across the street from us, who it turned out was a clarinetist with the NBC symphony orchestra, Jim Palmer. When my mom asked Mr. Palmer for help, he came up with this plan. I would make carbon copies of my homework. He would grade them and seal them in an NBC symphony official stationery envelope and write his name across the seals. We would save them and at the end of the term go to the administration with the collection.

Since my answers were all 100%, my nemesis was unmasked for the sick creature he was, and lost his job.

That wasn't the only occurrence. My homeroom teacher in seventh grade knew that I had to go to Hebrew Classes on certain evenings. Those were the only times I got detention! Conveniently only on those nights..... cute! And hard to prove too...

Bright spots

There were some bright spots in the whole school nightmare. At Tenafly Junior High, I became very close to Mr. Sol Feinstein, my photography teacher, and to a Mrs. Schiefele, on whom I guess I had a serious crush. I used to hang out at her class after my classes were over, and walk her to her car, carry her books, and so on.... I was crazy about her, and I think she knew it, and was at some level flattered. Later I would become close to a couple of High School teachers, like Clarence Graham, shop, and Richard Williams, who was never my teacher, but became the sponsor for the Photography Club at THS, which I started there..

After school was finished, I developed a real friendship and professional relationship with Mr. George Cameron, who was to become a really great influence on my life, and at the time his direction pushed me towards Biological sciences, and away from physical science.

Chemistry Class

When I got to my senior year I had not yet been able to take Chemistry, (largely because it was not offered until the senior year) to which of course I was really looking forward. I really expected become a Chemist, because I wanted to work with my dad in his pharmaceutical company. But the College Boards were given at the end of the Junior year, and I needed to take the Board in Chemistry for College. I took it anyway, and scored so high, that it left an impression on my would-be teacher when I began my senior classes and got "*Commander*" Warren Becht. It seems that Mr. Becht was pursuing an advanced degree at City College in New York, probably in "*torturing the Press family*", and had entered a very high level class in Chemical Kinetics, taught by none other than my cousin Jack Morrow.

Mr. Becht was not faring well in Jack's class, having apparently bitten off more than he could chew, and Jack politely asked him to withdraw. All of this unbeknownst at the time to poor me. Anyway he was the only Chemistry teacher at THS, and I had little choice. On the first day of class, after his introduction of the course, he made a special effort to intimidate me, coming right into my face as he told the class, "*by the way... I just want to tell you all, I don't hold your relatives against you*". This he certainly did.

Remember, when I began learning about Chemistry, I was only seven. That was ten years earlier, and before the International meeting known as IUPAC, which changed the official spelling of certain chemical names. So, when I was tested on things like "*Sulfate*", and "*Cloride*", I spelled them as I learned them "*Sulphate*" and "*Chloride*". Mr. Becht however, clearly aware of that, still chose to give me 0 credit for those answers. And, it didn't stop there.... On the final exam, there was some real cheating going on, but it wasn't mine.... Bottom line, by the time he finished with me, I was really turned off to Chemistry class. And, thus the influence of Mr. Cameron was really pivotal in my career direction.

Magic to Locksmithing

I also was into Magic tricks, and escape artistry. Dad and I loved to play "*tie me up*". A long clothes line and we could tie one another up, to see if we could escape, like Houdini. I got really good at it, and later wanted to be an escape artist. But, it would draw me into the world of locks and keys. I had a mentor in a neighbor. Ben Dalgin was an older gentleman, perhaps 70ish when I knew him. Mr. Dalgin was a member of the Society of American Magicians (SAM), in New York where Houdini had been their first President. At the time, I was too young to join the SAM, but there was another retiree who liked kids, and tried to get them interested in magic, named Arnold Belais. Arnold was a retired insurance agent, and organized the Independent Magical Performer's Society, or IMPS. We always joked that it was originally going to be called the Professional Independent Magical Performers Society, but ruled it out because of the initials.

National TV

Because of my magical interests, at age 13, I was asked to perform on *National* Television, on one of Merv Griffin's original TV shows called "*Play Your Hunch*". In this series, couples appeared as contestants and were entertained by three acts of some kind or other. One was a real one, and the others, fakes. I was the real Magician, and had to set up two other kids to start real tricks, but I was the only one who actually knew how to complete them. While waiting in the "*Blue Room*" backstage, I talked at length with Leon Uris, author of Exodus. Then when It was my turn, I took the tie from Merv's sidekick, Johnny Olsen, and cut it up. I loosened his shirt buttons and cuffs, and borrowed a bill from his wallet, promptly burning it to cinders, and then promising to restore the tie, the bill, and pull off his shirt without removing his jacket!

The money I got was to be dependent on whether the couples guessed that I was the real magician. They did pick me, but when asked, "why?" The couple that cost me the extra $50.00, said that removing someone's shirt without taking off their jacket was the only trick they had ever seen before. Imagine, I was cheated out of prize money because these yokels had never seen a magic show! In Tenafly though, I was quite the celebrity, for a short time, when I got back to classes the next day.

When I turned 17, the SAM changed their membership requirements and I was allowed to audition for membership. That meant performing a magical presentation at a meeting in front of some 300 magicians! Whew.... I finally made it on the second try. I became the youngest member Nationally in the SAM. And that had its perks too.... When the New York World's Fair was held in Flushing meadows in 1965, then National President Irving Desfor, took me up on the stage at the New York Power and Light Pavilion on the evening of "*SAM Day at the Fair*", and I was the one who turned on all the lights that evening. It was quite an honor.

After school, I used to wander around on Washington Ave. and after cruising through Frederick Harris' I'd stop at the Tenafly Paint and Glass store, a hardware store near the Junior High. Irv Fried, was the owner of the shop and we soon became friends, and I started to '*help out*" after school. Doing this had some real highlights, like when a little girl maybe 9 years old, came in and asked for some "*stolen wool*". I was probably a pain in the neck to him at first. But he taught me to cut (duplicate) keys, and I started to develop an interest in locks and locking devices. Eventually, I started a part-time business fixing locks, and even hung up a sign saying "*locksmith on premises*". I'd take in work, bring it home to my workshop, and bring it back again fixed in a couple of days. Irv liked the service and I made a few bucks. Soon I found Sonny Fisher in Englewood at Fisher's Housewares, and befriended his dad Sam, a glazier who bragged that he had "*glazed most of Englewood*".

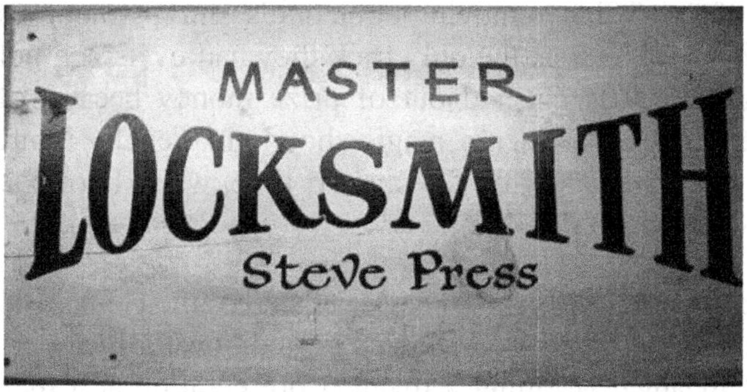

Fig 6. Locksmithing Sign

I posted a sign there too, and Sonny even gave me space for a workbench to change lock combinations on premises. Sam taught me to cut glass, and I liked the fact that there was a pet store next door too.

I'll never forget at about 14 years old, I was trying to learn where to buy parts for locks, and I foolishly went into the local locksmith's shop, "*Bill's*". Asking Bill to let me buy some "*pins and springs*" I was told "*I don't sell parts to competitors*". Wow, what a complement! And, how stupid! I was both pissed off, and psyched.

The whole security thing got really interesting to the point that when I graduated High School, since I was going to College at night anyway, I started up in earnest, though I took some vacations from this business to try working for others at various jobs for a few months at a time. Usually in chemically related fields.

Bill Oliveira

I worked variously for Mosa Havivi, a violin repairman and former cellist under Toscanini; then in Chemistry; variously at Washine Chemical Company, Pierre Le Doux, Penetone, Cilco Inks, and others. Finally, I found a sales job at Dictograph, and was privileged to be taught selling by a man named Bill Oliveira; a self made "*Fireball*" salesman. Bill would have another effect on my life, which he never knew about. It was Bill Oliveira who first told me about Chiropractic, telling me that he "*always wished he had become a Chiropractor instead.*"

But, finally, after leaving Dictograph, I settled back into the locksmithing business, and began dabbling in alarms as well. Naturally, being in that field, it paid for me to be close to the local police department, and I joined the Auxiliary Police and the Ambulance Corps as well.

My Sergeant, Bruce Ohlendorf, was the adopted son of then second in command in the Englewood Department, and a respected cop named Joe Ohlendorf. Everyone loved and respected. Joe. Bruce and I became good friends, and when he went to work for Rutger's University, teaching Civil Defense Courses under Federal grants, I got into all his courses and took that training. He also introduced me to Col. Carl Koenig, the County Civil Defense Coordinator, with whom I became good friends. It was Col Koenig, after whom the street where my kids now live is named, who sent me to Ossining, NY to study Radiation Health Physics at Lowell University, when I finished Chiropractic College.

Ambulances and Police

I really got into the emergency medicine thing, taking a MET (Medical Emergency Technician) Course in Haverstraw, NY and then the National registry exam for EMT's , passing it easily. Then I got into the first EMT class given in NJ as well, and took it all over again, as New Jersey stubbornly refused to give reciprocity to New York's class. So I was the first National Registry EMT in New Jersey aside from a few people who were "*grandfathered in*", who never took the test.

As things got going in this area, I was in on the ground floor. They had recently developed CPR at Johns-Hopkins and started teaching it to the "*lay Public*". Initially, it was only for Cardiologists! Then all Doctors, and finally they decided that everyone should or could learn it. I became the first non-physician to be accredited as an instructor in CPR too... then they formed a Bergen County Council of Emergency Medical Services. This was the nucleus of a movement to create what would become the Paramedic Program in Bergen County. And I was the Disaster Committee Chairman.

The Seed is Planted

It was during one of these meetings, that my future would be determined. I was terribly allergic as a kid, even going through seven years of injection treatments for the allergies, which were supposedly to ragweed, and other pollens, dust, animal dander etc. I was taking so many of a strong prescription anti-histamine, Ornade. Taking some six a day, I worried about poisoning as an effect of this addiction.

One evening, as our committee sat waiting for some members to show up, I was commiserating with Doctor Michael Jablonsky, who was at the time Chief of Medicine at Hackensack Hospital. When I told him about my allergies, he said, "*why don't you go to a Chiropractor?*". I was at that time studying Biochemistry at Fairleigh, so I kind of laughed... saying "*you're a medical doctor... why are you suggesting that? What can Chiropractic have to do with allergies*?". He said that he had had asthma as a child, and been regularly in *status asthmaticus*. His mother, in desperation, took him to a Chiropractor, and the asthmatic attacks stopped. He said it "*probably saved my life*". This left an indelible and accumulating effect on me.

So, one day, after getting into a couple of medical schools with a sort of "*early admission*", I was talking to one of my lab instructors at Fairleigh, Dr. Sion Daftari . Sion suggested that he could arrange an interview for me with Dr. Ernest Napolitano, then President of what was at the time still called Columbia Institute of Chiropractic. I went to the interview and was almost immediately accepted. When I started classes, they were in the process of changing their name to New York Chiropractic College, because they wanted accreditation from the New York Board of regents, and there was an obvious conflict with Columbia University's name. Anyway, the rest is history.

Skating gets into my blood

It was not to be until I graduated High School that I got voluntarily into sports. In fact, until then I so detested sports that I even went to Summer Camps that catered to science nerds. One day this would prove embarrassing. After High School, I asked a girl named Grace Carrino for a date , and she told me she was "*going to Roller Skate on Saturday*". I could come along. When the session ended, there were enough dance skaters to warrant organizing a "*Dance Special*", besides it was a kind of commercial for the Pros there, Andy and Mary Lisovsky, who had been champion skaters in the 30's and 40's.

With the usual teenage male braggadocio, I told Grace, whom I never saw again, that "*I will compete against those guys in a year*". I got really hooked. I went out Monday morning and bought my own skates, and began skating some 40 hours a week for years after that. I can still recall my mother's horror when she heard that I spent about $300.00 for skates… she must have thought I was completely mad. Finally the end of that year, I did in fact compete, and win, against some of the dancers that skated that afternoon. The skating was also a social outlet. There were lots of pretty girls there, and many male skaters aren't interested in girls, so there was less competition in that department. I loved it, and started winning competitions, initially with Darella "*Dee*" Parliman, and later with Linda Ackerman, grand-daughter of the rink's organist.

A Day With the Champ

During the same period, and due to my interest in magic, I found myself one afternoon in Manhattan. Actually, I was supposed to be delivering printed goods for my mother, who was, at that time, running my father's business affairs.

Walking down Broadway, near 42nd St., I passed a store I had frequented many times as a younger kid. It was a penny arcade, but with an entire section devoted to selling magic tricks.

A crowd had gathered in front, and knowing the shop well, I was able to get into the front of the crowd, through the other door and back outside. Who should I spy standing and staring into the window at the magical paraphernalia but Mohammed Ali.

Realizing that he was interested in magic, I trotted right up to the famous man, and showing him my Society of American Magician's Card, I inquired as to whether he was interested in magic? He told me he was, so I suggested that the stuff they sold at this shop was mass marketed equipment, and I could show him where the pros get their stuff. In his inimitable way, he asked me "*would you really do that for me*?" And, we walked together to his waiting car.

He was traveling with a friend, another really big guy, who probably owned the purple El dorado we got into. I understand that the friend was a radio announcer from the Carolinas. I took them only a few blocks, but the trip was really memorable, not only because I was so crammed into the front seat with "*the Greatest*", but that he and his friend were SO big that I was that squeezed in even in the capacious front set of an El dorado Cadillac! The Champ was not even sitting straight front, but sideways the whole trip, waving to admiring fans all the way.

We soon arrived at Lou Tannen's, where Lou had already retired and his brother Mel was still running the shop. I was still a regular at Tannen's in that period, and when I introduced Mel to the Champ, I became an instant VIP at the store. We were shown to a back room where Mel arranged to demonstrate real professional illusions for Mr. Ali and myself.... The wonderment on Ali's face at each trick was marvelous to behold, and I was able to ask him more about this "*hobby*".

It seems that he had recently lost his boxing license due to the draft evasion scandal. And, he was thinking what to do with his career. If the draft issue had kept him from continuing to box, he was preparing to reinvent himself as a stage illusionist!

Later, he was reputed to have been booted from the British Magical Association for allegedly revealing the secret to a coveted trick there.

We were together that day so long, I began to feel we had become friends, so I invited the Champ to come to my parents home for dinner.... It was only a short time after the release of the Sidney Poitier movie "G*uess who's coming to dinner?",* and I enjoyed being able to say that to my rather surprised mother.... Unfortunately Mr. Ali never made it to Tenafly.

Chapter 2

Better to Have Loved and Lost

**

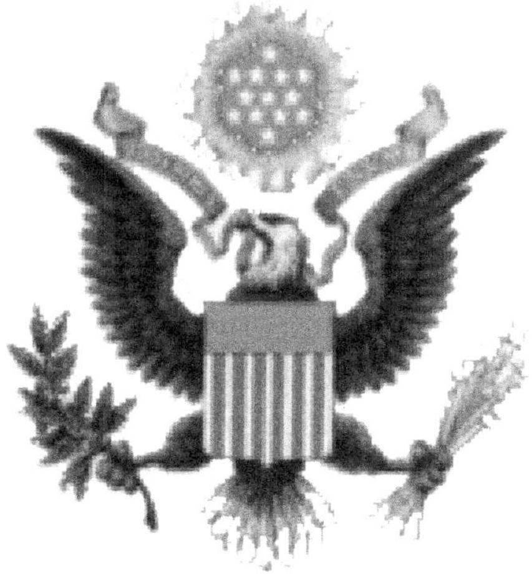

I was only 23 when I met JoAnn. She was 17. We met while skating at Paramus Roller Rink. It was 1970. JoAnn was until that time, the sweetest girl I had ever met. Her high intellect shone through her dark Sicilian eyes, and I was smitten. She too was in love. When she told her dad that I played the cello, spoke French and had my own business (locksmith), they didn't believe her. Finally, her dad told her she could date me if "*I could show up with a cello and actually play something*" I did, and we dated.

My Adult Life Begins

One needs to take into account that JoAnn was still in High School. Though since she was an exceptional student, she had taken extra credit classes each semester, and we calculated that she could skip her Senior year and still graduate.

Eventually she told her parents that she wanted to marry me. Naturally they were horrified that their little girl was contemplating marriage at such a young age. They had such plans for her after all. She was forbidden to marry. We, of course, had other ideas.

One evening JoAnn told me that she "*thought*" she "*was pregnant*". Without batting an eyelash, I told her that I loved her and that we "*should get married*". That was when she told her parents, only that she wanted to marry, of course. When they forbade her to marry me, we hatched a plot.

The Elopement

The next evening we saw each other, we concocted a plan to elope. Her parents both worked. So, one morning she would leave ostensibly for school, and I would be waiting around the corner for her. She had secretly packed all her things the night before, but left them in her closet, hidden from view.

After leaving, she came to me and we waited for her mom to leave. JoAnn returned surreptitiously to the house, and retrieved her things, ALL her things... cleaning out her room. We left for our wedding.

But how could we wed when she was still underage and needed parental consent? I researched the rules for obtaining a marriage license, and found that one could show any proof of age, including a baptismal record. So, when we looked through all her documents to find something we could alter, we found her baptismal record form, where the date was hand written and did alter it. It worked, and we got the license, so when the appointed day came, and we ran off, we were armed with the proper (sort of) documents. Still, we had no idea who we could get to do the ceremony.

A Church Wedding

We headed into the "*Big Apple*", and after cruising around a bit, found an Episcopal Church which was open. There a willing and understanding Priest officiated, pronouncing us man and wife. We found a room at the Holiday Inn in midtown and waited until the next day to call her folks.

In retrospect what we did to them was probably too cruel. But with their prohibition, and in our youthful zeal, we felt our hands tied. Besides, I knew they were good Catholics and would never consent to an abortion if it were their decision to make. But now as Husband and Wife we could make that decision together. We were really both too young to become parents. Such things were still not legal in New Jersey, but in New York one could obtain a "*therapeutic abortion*" on demand at any hospital.

I certainly did not marry JoAnn just because she was pregnant. And by the way, I was never too sure that she really was. Of course, by the time we could arrange the procedure, there was no longer much doubt, since once we determined to go through with it, there was no longer any reason to take precautions. Thus if she wasn't pregnant when she told me she was, she certainly was when she entered the Hospital.

If JoAnn used a phony pregnancy to trap me into marrying her, it was unnecessary, and I really still believe it was not a conscious ploy. I knew she was a really good person, unselfish to a tee, and so very bright. I was fully prepared to marry her regardless.

Her Parents Relent

When they realized that we were this serious, her parents decided that they didn't want their mistake to cost her a real wedding, so they arranged for us to be "*re-married*" in a ceremony at a lovely catering hall in Garfield called the Villa Roma. I always adored her folks despite their few foibles.

Her School Days Come Back to Haunt Us

The Viet Nam War was raging, and I was fighting to keep my student deferment. While all the time attending College at night, I operated my own business as a Locksmith and Alarm Systems Designer and Installer during the day.

This was a business I started while still in High School, and it gave me a fair living. So, when I needed to find us a place to start our lives, I was able to pay the rent on a modest garden apartment in Englewood.

JoAnn came to work with me in the office, learned to cut keys and ran the shop while I went out on calls. One day, I came back to find her sobbing and bleeding from the scalp. She had failed to head my warning to put her hair up and caught a lock of her waist length hair in the key machine, which instantly yanked it completely out… ! She quickly recovered and life went on.... I thought we were both very happy.

It wasn't long before JoAnn longed to get a college degree. Earlier that June, her High School Class graduation ceremony was held. Though she wasn't there, her name was called, they even used her married name... "*JoAnn Press*" they called out; and the entire graduating class bore witness. A girlfriend offered to bring her the diploma and was given the certificate in her place. When we received the diploma, it was clear, she had graduated from Memorial High School in what was then still called East Paterson, NJ; even though she had not been present her entire last year of school.

So, JoAnn enrolled at Bergen Community to take a degree in accounting. Right off, we were told that she needed a High School Diploma to matriculate, and when she showed them her East Paterson Diploma they enrolled her.

The Mid-Term

She took Accounting courses, and in her second year was required to take Intermediate Accounting. I understand this is the class which separates the Accountants from the Bookkeepers. She came home after the Mid-term in tears. She wailed... "*I failed it, I failed it...*" totally inconsolable.....still I tried.... I said, *"what does that mean, You failed? Got a "B"?"*. I thought she'd at least smile, but nothing... she really thought she had failed a test, probably for the first time in her life.

Two weeks later, she came back from class with a smile from ear to ear. I knew..... I asked her "*so, you Aced the test after all*?" "*yeah....*" She said sheepishly. "*So tell me?*" I demanded.... "*well*" she went on.... *"The professor knew that the test was too hard for anyone to Ace it, so he added 16 extra points."....* I prodded on.... "*So, what was your score?"* ..... she hesitated to tell me...... "*116*" !

Anyway, after a while, she needed to transfer to a four-year college, and when she tried to enter Fairleigh Dickinson University, we were told that they needed her transcript to enroll her for a degree. When they got the transcript, East Paterson had stubbornly refused to indicate that they had graduated her, despite giving out her diploma at graduation. We should have sued them.

The High School Fails

I called the School to inquire what kind of snafu had occurred? There was a woman Vice-Principal, Mrs…something, and the Principal was one Dr. Vito Farese. I spoke to the Vice-principal who informed that "*her transcript indicated that she had not graduated*".

At the time, I was serving Englewood as Director of Civil Defense and Disaster Control, and Chief of Auxiliary Police, and was sitting in my office at City Hall when I called. Frankly I was expecting a little credibility for my position. However, the Vice-Principal asked me if I would come to the School and show her the diploma, so "*we could clear up the mix-up.*"

Smelling a rat, and fearful of a plan to take it away from us, I had the diploma framed, so no one could easily tear it from my hands and rip it up. When Jo and I got to the school, the Vice-principal told me she "*needed to make a photo-copy, so could I remove it from the frame please?*" I told her that it "*would copy just fine in the frame, but the frame wasn't going to leave my hands for a second*". She was visibly shaken at her failure to steal back the diploma. After we copied it, she admitted that it was genuine. But insisted that JoAnn had not graduated from their High School.

I'm Threatened

The next day I got an irate call from a "Dr" Farese. It went something like this:

Farese: *Hello Mr Press?*

Me: *Yes*

Farese: *This is Doctor Farese, the Principal at East Paterson Memorial High School*

Me: *Yes, how can I help you?*

Farese: *I WANT that diploma*

Me: *I beg your pardon??*

Farese: *I don't know how you got our diploma, but I want it back*

Me: *Listen, Mr Farese…*

Farese: *That's Doctor Farese….*

Me: *When you act like a Doctor, I'll treat you like a Doctor…*

I take umbrage at the idea that this diploma was not issued by your administration. What are you implying?

Farese: *I'm just saying that someone, somehow got hold of a Diploma blank, and wrote her name on it, because we didn't issue that diploma*

Me *You will NEVER get that diploma back because JoAnn graduated fair and square, and there are over a hundred witnesses that she did.*

Farese: *Well then I may have to go to the authorities to retrieve it.*

Me: *I suggest you do what you have to do, and we'll do what we have to do. Good bye.*

PS – we never heard from the likes of him again. But, they never did give her the change in transcript to go with the diploma.

Gets Two Diplomas

Regardless, the school refused to confirm to Fairleigh that JoAnn graduated, so we did some more research and found out that the State has a program for people who never finish High School, in which, if they enroll in Community College as non-matriculants and attain a minimum of 25 credits with a C average (JoAnn was straight A student), they will give you a GED (General Equivalency Diploma) without taking the GED Exam.

She got her GED and had the High School Diploma too and was enrolled in FDU.

Shortly afterwards, Jo began to pack on the pounds. She knew that her appearance was important to me, and still despite our love for one another, she got heavier and heavier. Eventually topping 250 pounds on her 5'6" frame. Still I didn't leave. By then she was working for Volkswagen of America in Englewood Cliffs, and was rising rapidly through their ranks as she progressed in College. They saw her intellect despite the exterior and put it to good use, treating her very well. She quickly rose from Clerk-typist, to Accountant.

Meanwhile I was enrolled in what was Columbia Institute of Chiropractic, in Manhattan, but changed its name to New York Chiropractic College, and moved in time for me to start in Long Island, at the campus of New York Institute of Technology, in Glen Head.

New York was trying to completely revamp their programs to keep pace with the requirements of New York State Board of Regents Accreditation, which was a do or die proposition for them. The Council on Chiropractic Education (CCE) had just been recognized by the US Dept of Education, and Chiropractic Colleges all over the Country had to get rid of their faculty full of DC's who were taught by DC's *ad nauseum*. This was known as an inbred education, and it had to stop. All they could teach now were specific techniques courses. All the Sciences had to have Scientists teaching them.

Well it turned out that NYCC was in a good location to get the best Professors who would moonlight from their jobs at the top Medical Schools in the New York area. We had Biochemistry with a Biochemistry Professor from Albert Einstein, Microbiology from Mt Sinai, etc….. we had taken a quantum leap into the 20th Century for Chiropractic.

I had been involved in the local City emergency services for some years by this time, having served on the Ambulance corps, the Auxiliary Police and the Red Cross Disaster Team. I chaired the Red Cross Team, became the first non doctor to be certified in CPR as an instructor in New Jersey, and was the first person the take and pass the National Registry for EMT's in the State as well. When I started in NYCC, I was named by Mayor Walter Taylor to the position of Director of the City's Civil Defense and Disaster Corps, making me Chief of Auxiliary Police, Auxiliary Fire and the Radio Amateur Civil Emergency Service (RACES).. I had a red light and siren in my Volkswagen bug, and a bronze plaque in the back to bear witness to this prestigious position. Unfortunately it said, "Director CD-DC".

A Vice-President of NYCC, who must have been a frustrated cop. He saw the plaque and immediately hated me. He used the DC business to complain that I "*had no right to be a director of DC's, when I wasn't yet a DC*" (Doctor of Chiropractic). It meant only Disaster Control, but he didn't care, and plotted to boot me from NYCC.

Although I could have stayed and been under this nut's thumb the rest of my schooling. Palmer College had an established Clinic anyway, and at NYCC, the burden of building a clinical practice would have been mine as they had just opened. It was under these circumstances that I applied to other Chiropractic Colleges, and got into Palmer, another accredited College, and the place it all began. Had that lunatic been successful in throwing me out, I would have been forced to go to Atlanta, to Life College, which was at that time, taking any and everyone at that time, as it was not yet accredited.

So, when my acceptance came through at Palmer, I jumped at the opportunity, and packed my bags.

Refuses To Go To Iowa

When I arrived at Palmer, it was a really impressive place. They had been in operation for 75 years & had a reputation, and an enormous variety of cases in the clinic. My clinical experience would be that much richer there, although a consequence of transferring was then that Colleges didn't accept one another's technique courses, so I had to take additional classes to catch up to my classmates at Palmer... thus I have trained twice as much in techniques as the rest of my classmates with whom I started at NYCC.

JoAnn refused to accompany me there. And, considering her refusal to anything about her now gross obesity, I guess I was to some extent relieved. Still I loved her and longed for my cute little girl back.

Don't Come Home

The next Christmas Holiday, on a call home, I was telling her that I'll be home in two days, and she simply said "*Don't come home*". She had had an affair with some 6'4", 250lb African-American guy she met at the Rink, named "*Calvin*". She later told me that she just assumed that I would never take her back after that. I never asked for an explanation of that reasoning. And, considering her psychological issues, that was probably the reason she did it.

We went together to a lawyer and got a no-fault divorce. I was both relieved and heart-broken.

How To Destroy Your Child's Psyche

It turns out that around age nine, JoAnn's dad, who apart from this huge faux pas, was always a really nice guy, ... got mad about something, and just losing momentary control, yelled at her one day.... "*You were an accident, and are to be seen around here and not heard from.... You are just tolerated here....*" It broke her self esteem and set her on a course of self-hatred and self destruction, which culminated in our split; but not for obvious reasons.

It would not be until years later when she finally got away from "*Calvin*", who was cheating on her, and even made her sick.... and got under counseling, that she discovered what made her tick.

Self Loathing

At a lunch some years later, she admitted to me that it came out in her counseling sessions that she was "*so filled with self-loathing and loved me so much*", that she "*couldn't imagine the man she loved spending his life with the likes of her*". And had thereby set upon a course of self destruction, for the purpose of subconsciously driving me away so I could be really happy. What she didn't take into account was that I WAS really happy with her. I just wanted the old JoAnn back, but that JoAnn was irretrievably lost to me now.

Happy Ending

After many more years, I saw her again, at the funeral of an Aunt who had insulted me with an anti-semitic remark when we were still married. I went, not for the aunt, but to see Jo and her family and be there for these good people I still care about.

JoAnn was there with her new husband, and had slimmed down to a semblance of normalcy and really looked good. Moreover they had recently had a child together, and seemed really happy. She introduced me to her Husband, and I told him to "*take really good care of her*"... He said "*I will, why?*" I told him "*because you are lucky enough to be with the best woman on Earth*". She cried.... Happy tears.

I truly wish them all the best and all the happiness I could not give her years earlier.

Chapter 3

The License Arrives!

**

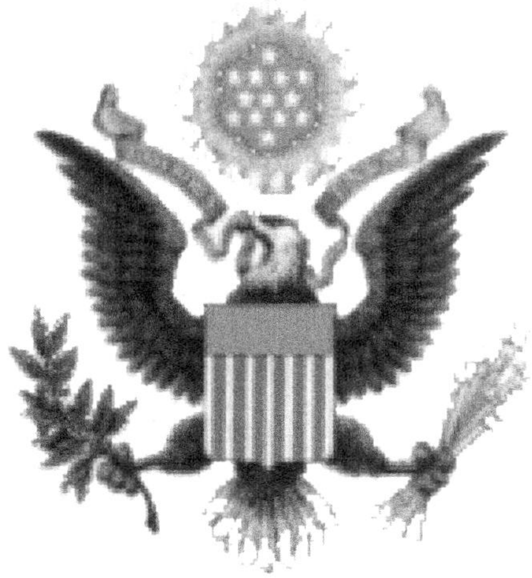

When I applied to New York Chiropractic College, it was, as I have already explained, still called Columbia Institute of Chiropractic, but by the time I started there, they had changed the name to NYCC. I still needed to earn some money on the side, and I decided to continue installing alarm systems.

Cheating a Colleague

One day I was passing the office of a colleague in Englewood whose name sounded perfect for a Chiropractor, and I just thought I'd say "*hi*" to someone with whom I expected to one day soon have a professional relationship. We'll call him Dr. "*Spine*". There were two of them, a father & son. The dad had entered Chiropractic college after his son graduated and they seemed to be in some kind of partnership. Push came to shove and we talked about what I was doing for a living. When I mentioned that I installed security systems, the son told me that they needed an alarm for their clinic. Seeing an opportunity to develop a friendship, I gave them a very good price. About 35% below market at that time. Son grabs the deal, and I arrange to install the system. When I finish installing what he bought, and come to collect the balance of my fee, he tells me that they decided they need another window done, so I come back to add that on to the contract.

Finished again, I ask for my funds. This time, I'm told by son that only dad has the checkbook and I'll have to come back another day. Ok, I start to smell a rat, but I swallow my pride and come back on the appointed day. This time Dad has reasons why my installation is sub-par… now understand that I was doing this for a living for the previous nine years, and was professionally trained; his complaints were not founded in fact. It was just stall tactics, and I knew it. But it gave me a pretext to go to the closet where the equipment was installed, i.e., the alarm panel and dialer (together, worth more than the balance due.) I loosened the wiring harness and mounting screws preparing to repossess the equipment if I were not paid. Had I been paid, I would have gone back and tightened up everything to "*double check the system*". Dad tells me that he's "*not prepared to pay me*" what he owes me, and I should "*just count myself lucky that I got the deposit*". I.e., theft by deception. I was serving as Chief of Auxiliary Police in the same town and had the power of arrest with my shield in pocket.

I said nothing. I simply went past the closet, took the panels off the wall, placed them under my arm, and started out the door. Dad, a little guy; maybe 60-ish, came running after me yelling "*put that back or I'll get my gun and blow your head off*". I stepped back and showed him my shield, saying "*one step backwards and your career is over*". "*I am about to arrest you for theft by deception, terroristic threats and if you take another step, for assault with a deadly weapon as well*". He stopped in his tracks, but yelled at me as I left.... "*just try to get a license in New Jersey. I am on the Licensing board's committee on ethics, and you will never get licensed in this state*".

It was with this kind of cloud hanging over my head that I spent the next three plus years and finished Chiropractic school. I have already described the brouhaha I had at New York Chiropractic College with a zealous, jealous official there. So, when I finally took and passed my licensing exam, an enormous weight was finally off not only me, but my parents too....

When the license arrived via the nice African-American letter-carrier in Tenafly, I imagine he was rather surprised to get kissed by my mother when she saw that large envelope from the Board of Medical Examiners.

I really wanted to file suit against that SOB, but my dad made me promise never to do so, to just let it rest. I dutifully obeyed. I still harbor a deep distaste for this immoral man with a DC degree.

Locksmithing again

Patty also tried to be a good wife, and the relationship started out really well. She's a decent person, if not the most brilliant girl in the world, and aside from the moral issues which kept me from starting a family with her, in retrospect, I probably could have been happy with Patty. In the beginning, when I was struggling the first time around to develop a practice, she was working as an accountant, but even together the income wasn't enough to cover the bills. My parents subsidized us for a while, and after several months, my Dad got tired of the subsidy.... He came to me and suggested that as I was "*only seeing patients on Monday, Wednesday and Friday*", that it seemed to him that I was therefore just free on the other days... so, "*what are you doing on those days?*" he'd ask.... I tried to explain that I was out trying to meet people, hand out cards and build the practice... but he insisted that I try to take a part-time job despite my explanations that I might be away and miss a new patient, which would "*cost me more than the amount I could make in salary for a three-day-a-week part-time job*".

Unconvinced, he pressured me to go back to locksmithing, as I was a master locksmith after all. So, I finally acceded to his pressure and went into the City and took a spot for twelve dollars an hour. Trudging into the City with my toolbox, in old clothes, I started at a lock shop on the lower east side.

The first job I was given was to open a van from which the owner was locked out. So I took the boss' van and drove the customer to some corner, and got on my knees to pick the lock. While sitting there, an elderly Jewish man came over and was standing over me watching intently what I was doing and how I comported myself. As I opened the door, I looked up to see who it was, and he just stared at my face and said..*"so vat are ye dooink dis for? Ya oughtta be a dockta!"*... I couldn't even answer. I had had it as a locksmith.

Johns-Hopkins

While still at New York Chiropractic College, I got a brochure in the mail, from Johns-Hopkins College of Medicine in Baltimore, offering a class in Trauma, medical and Surgical Emergencies. Being an EMT and interested in advancing my knowledge generally in the field, I determined to go.

The course was divided into three "*tracks*". One for EMT's, one for Nurses, and one for Physicians. When I arrived in Baltimore, I registered and started in the class for EMT's where I had registered. But, soon I was wandering over to the Physician's table and looking at their curriculum. Finally I got up the nerve to ask someone if it really made a difference which track I took, and was told to ask the director, who okayed my transfer.

That day at lunch, I was sitting across the table from an elderly doctor dressed in a white lab coat with all the doctor accoutrements. Engaging him in conversation, we got to a point where he asked me what kind of doctor I was. When I told him Chiropractic, he said *"a Chiropractor? What are you doing here?"*. I simply indicated that I was also an EMT and had come that route, but wanted to further my education. However, I had picked up a brochure about a forthcoming program that was much more intense; a "*first postgraduate course in the pathology of bone and joints*", to be held only for board certified orthopedists, radiologists, and pathologists. They weren't even admitting their own residents!

So, then he asked me, *"but you guys don't believe in the germ theory of disease do you?"* He actually thought we never heard of germs! I told him, we certainly do study the germ theory, but perhaps we interpret it differently that he did. This piqued his interest and he asked me what I meant?... I said, well, you know "[3]*Koch's postulates*". He naturally had. I went on..... "*well, I simply don't think that that goes far enough! If you take a culture of an organism and inject it into a healthy animal, then all you have proven is that when an animal has that disease, then that organism is going to be present in its system. But, by inoculating it with billions of germs in a massive injection, you have only shown that you can overload its immune system in an unnatural way.*"... He looked at me and said, "*you know, I never thought about it like that*".

Then he noticed the brochure for the bone and joint course, and thinking he was torturing me, he said, "*I'll bet you'd like to go to that course?*". I said, "*of course I would, it's right in my own field. That would be great*!".... he handed me his card and said, "*send your application to my attention. I'll see you are admitted*". Wow... this was George Zuidema, the surgeon-in-chief of Johns-Hopkins Hospital.

London

The year I married Stephanie, we spent a vacation at a Jewish resort in the Catskills at a place called "*the Brown's*". I had been there several times and gotten to know Charles and Lillian Brown, the owners. So, I had really good seats in the "*Brown Derby Lounge*" one evening when London Lee was entertaining.

He was a smash hit, and had us all rolling in the isles laughing. London Lee was the scion of the founder of

---

[3] Dr. Koch, the developed of a TB Vaccine, had written that the way to discern if a germ is the cause of a specific disease, is to take a test animal, and infect it with a culture of organisms grown in medium and then observe that animal to see if it develops the infection. If so, then you have proven that that organism is the cause of the disease.

Kimberly Knits, and one of the few, if not the sole comedian in the business who came not from poverty, but from wealth.

His routine made the most of that with lines like… "*my father was so rich, I was Bar Mitzvah…. In the Vatican*". London, it turned out was living in Alpine, about ten minutes from my office and was looking for a Chiropractor. We became fast friends. I was invited to accompany him on tour, and attended all his shows in the area. He even coached me on timing and delivery and vastly improved the way I tell jokes. Thus we would trade stories while sitting in the care on the way to his "*gigs*".

Vito and the wise guys

One evening, he showed up in front of the office in a new Mercedes S Class. Calling to me to come out, I came to the window. He tells me "*your're driving*". I hesitated, having never driven such a car before. I asked whose car was this? He turned around and introduced me to Vito and Marie… Genovese, Jr !!!

We drive uneventfully to the Pocmont somewhere in the Poconos, and are given, thanks to the presence of Vito and the Mrs., a table right at the stage.

During the drive, London was having one of his anxiety attacks and I trying to calm him down, tell him… "*London, you're a professional…. As soon as you get into your shtick, you'll be fine…*".. He answers " *I'll show you what anxiety is all about*". I said… "*what do you mean?*". He continues… "*I'm calling you on stage so YOU can be funny!*"

Hoping against hope that he might actually do that, I dared him…. Saying "*you wouldn't dare!*".

My Debut

Middle of the show, he says to the audience, "*Ladies and Gentlemen, it gives me great pleasure to introduce an up and coming but unknown young Comedian, Dr Stephen Press.*".... the audience starts clapping and I'm showing him my palms, trying to say "no"... Then Vito says to me.... "*geddup on the stage*!".... I got up on the stage. I actually don't even remember the stairs.

Frankly, I was never stage-shy, and had a few lines to use... some written by London, and a few others I had prepared in my mind while I was listening to the show, in case he did this. When I was facing London, in front of some 3000 people, he sticks the microphone in my face, and says "*ok, now YOU be funny*!" oops! I was prepared .... never lost my cool and got laugh after laugh. After five or six minutes.... I stuck the microphone back in his face and said, "*ok, London, had enough*?" The audience, realizing what had just happened, roared. During the ensuing intermission, they came and asked for my autograph. I took out business cards and signed the back of them.

The next real hint of possible trouble with this relationship came one day when he tells me that I have to see his friend and the "*godfather to his children*". Warren G, who was a high ranking official in the teamsters union, remember the year.... It was 1980.... Hoffa time ! We drive to the Bronx, where I am greeted by this classical wise-guy type. It turns out his neck is in pain, and I am the one to fix him up. Vito was in the back of the room, and when I took Warren's head in my hands to adjust him, Vito says "*does he know what he's got in his hands?*". Gulp.

There was talk about having me run a panel for the Teamsters Welfare Fund, reviewing Chiropractic Claims. About a week later, I get a call from London, telling me that Vito and Warren and he are "*going to Platos' retreat, with a couple of Massage Therapists from Vito's chain of Massage therapy centers, and"* they wanted me *"to come along"*. I was both thrilled and scared. Though I had been there before, it was with Patty, and they didn't know that. Stephanie was by then six months pregnant with Bobby, and I was not about to give these guys the power over my marriage that this would have given them. I demurred and the entire discussion of the welfare panel evaporated.

Shortly after that I never saw London again either. Strange.... Draw your own conclusions.

Bogotà

Through my sports medicine connections, I met many interesting people. At one American College of Sports Medicine Congress, I became friendly with a guy who turned out to be an official in Buenos Aires, in their Sports Ministry. One day he calls me and tells me that he has told the President of the professional football (soccer) team Santa Fe, in Bogotà, Colombia that I can be helpful to them. He arranged a contract between their President Señor Pachon-Roncancio and I, to treat the athletes, fit them with orthotics, take body fat measurements, and make prescriptions for their fitness.

I am to be paid some twenty-two thousand dollars, plus round trip first class travel for me, and coach for two of my staff. I take one young lady who was working for me who was herself Colombian, and a young man, who was working with the orthotics company.

We arrive, in Bogotà two days after the raid by terrorists on the Supreme Court in which the Seven Supreme Court Justices were murdered. Terrorism in Bogotà was rampant. On arrival, I am told that we will go nowhere without an armed escort! Our guards have submachine guns.

I work with their athletes, and really enjoy the time there. Despite that one evening while I was in our hotel, a bomb went off down the street at the Hotel Tecandamo, in the casino. Such fun!

One evening as we were being entertained at the Lido de Paris night club, Sr. Roncancio tells me in heavily accented English… *"you know, Dr Press, this is very espensive for me, and I am very **pure**"*. I giggled a little, and said, "*Sr. Roncancio, no creeo*" (I don't believe you)…. He started to get hot under the collar and protesting his honesty, told me "*I'm not a liar*"…. I just smiled and explained that in English, "*pure*" means "*puro*", and "*poor*" is "*pobre*"…. So, I continued, "*Pobre puede, puro no creeo*!"…. He had told me that he was a Virgin,when he meant to tell me he was poor. We all laughed…. Little did I realize that he was not a liar but would turn out to be a thief.

I performed all my agreed upon tasks, and Roncancio at the last day, hands me a couple of thousand more dollars telling me that I'll get the rest, (some $12,000 due) through the mail. I was tempted to take the orthotics with me home, and send them when I got payment, but something foolishly told me to trust this guy. Naturally I was stiffed. I complained to the Colombian Embassy, in Washington, but they never lifted a finger to help me. Oh well, at least I didn't lose money, and had a nice vacation in beautiful downtown Bogotà.

Chapter 4

Great Love, Great Tragedy

**

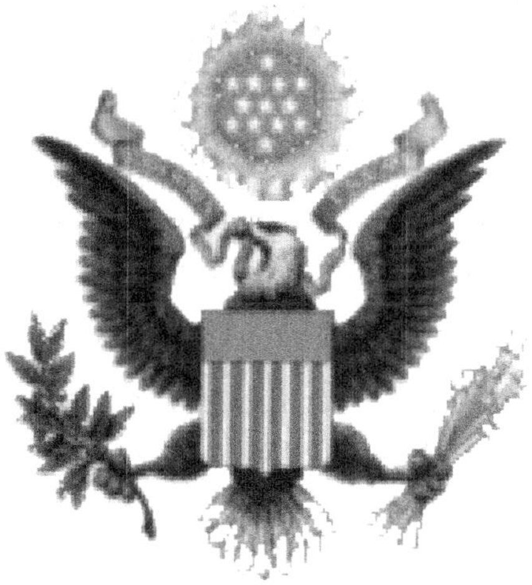

The greatest tragedy of my life, and the one thing for which I have real, and deep regrets, is the outcome of my love affair with Pascale. It all began when I was married to my second wife, Patty. Patty was bisexual, and although it was a stupid male ego thing to marry her, thinking we could share other women, and still maintain a relationship, I did make that mistake, failing miserably to listen to my inner voice. We were together only three years, and had no children together, but still, it was another trauma to part when we finally realized that it couldn't work like that.

Plato's

Remember that there was no such thing as AIDS and the worst thing one could get under normal circumstances was Syphilis or Gonorrhea, both still easily treatable with antibiotics. Most women were taking "*the pill*", and sex was far more open and natural than now. Meanwhile, life with Patty goes on.... and some of it was really interesting and daring, even risqué... there had been a few evenings at the infamous Plato's retreat in the Big Apple, and a fling with a mutual friend. But when Pascale came to stay the Summer, a new chapter in my life opened, and it would take many years to get past it.

One must realize that under the circumstances of my rather "*open*" relationship with Patty, we didn't consider it "*cheating*" for me to cultivate a liaison with another woman, so long as the motivation was ultimately to share her with Patty.

After several seasons of hosting foreign exchange students, mostly from France, with whom no liaisons had even been entertained, Pascale showed up at our door early one Summer. Patty and I went to greet her.... Pascale was just18, I was 34.

When the door opened, I could feel an electricity I have felt only one other time in my life. With my beloved Olga.

Dyspnea

It was hard to breathe. I didn't eat or sleep well the next few days, and knew I was smitten. Pascale was blonde, with hair of smoothest silk, and golden eyes, of a hue I have never seen before or since. She was petite, and built slender and solid. I would later find out she had been a gymnast of national class in France.

Patty at once knew that this was a girl who would be attractive to both of us. The question she had was whether I could bring her to our bed, then transition the affair to a ménage-a-trois. This latter was never to occur. And that was part of the demise of the marriage with Patty, though in no sense to be blamed on Pascale.

The seduction began almost from the onset, though it is hard now to say with any sense of objectivity, who was seducing whom. There was to be a US Olympic Festival in Syracuse that Summer, and I needed to go there for career reasons. Patty and I discussed it, and I invited Pascale to go along. I wanted her, but it was too dangerous to make any overt move towards this young (though legally adult) charge. Still the desire for her was overwhelming. We checked, still innocently, into a motel, and had separate beds, maintaining our respective privacy. But in the middle of the night, I was dreaming about how to approach her, and when I saw her lying asleep in the next bed, barely covered by a sheet, I was overcome by desire. Despite these feelings, I made no move to touch this sleeping angel.

Later, we visited an art museum, and when given a chance, she leaned over a railing, knowing me to be standing behind her, and rather obviously held her gorgeous dérriere in a pose that invited a touch. She was now obviously soliciting my attentions. Still, I resisted. On another evening, we went to Windows on the World, the restaurant at the 107th floor of the World Trade Center tower, and stood together, looking out under the stars on the clearest of nights, able to see over all New York City. It was like standing in a stationary airplane. The romance of the place led to a first kiss, and, though fleeting, it was deeply meaningful to me. I was in love with her.

After leaving Windows on the World, and having kissed, we went to the Palisades to enjoy another romantic view, and there, in the privacy of the darkness, we embraced and kissed one another with all the passion that our mutual desire could generate. We were now star-crossed lovers, though we had not yet consummated that love.

Naturally I couldn't tell Patty I was in love with Pascale, so if I was ever dishonest with a spouse, it was keeping this secret. When I advised Patty that I knew Pascale wanted me too, she arranged to go to friends in the Hamptons so we could have a week alone in the house. It was not long before Pascale and I consummated our love, and her relative innocence was an ever greater basis of arousal for me. Though she admitted she was not a virgin when we met, she had only a very limited encounter with a boy at a "*camping*", and was still very, very shy and innocent in every way. It took a lot of explaining to make her understand why Patty had permitted us to stay home alone, and why it would be ok for us to be intimate together. And, I never actually told her that Patty wanted to join us in the same bed. I instinctively knew she would never consent to that, and because I loved her, though I really had no right to, I wanted to continue our affair as long as possible, though at that moment, despite the depth of my feelings, I was not prepared to divorce Patty just yet, despite beginning to entertain those ideas.

The Wife Returns Home

Finally, (it seemed only a few hours, but was more than a week), Patty arrived home. And, as so many women seem to be capable of, she at once smelled that something more than a simple seduction was in the air. When I made it clear that Pascale and I had been together, she demanded that I arrange a ménage-a-trois, and when I was unable to accommodate her demands, she entered into a tirade.

Sweet little Pascale unable to fully comprehend the basis of the complex and perhaps strange "*New York Scene*" sexual mores, asked my mother to allow her to stay at their home (my parents) for the balance of her stay in the States.

Alarm Bells

With the clarity of thought which sometimes comes from 20-20 hindsight, I now know what transpired after she left my bed and board. It appears that when my mother asked her why she wanted to move to them, instead of staying with me, Pascale not able to tell my mother, that she was "*sleeping with your son, and despite having her permission, his wife got angry*", simply told her what she thought was an innocent white lie, and just said, "*Stephen was coming on to me, and I was uncomfortable with it*". My mother, who had only recently financially helped subsidize the launch of my career, saw red flags, and heard alarm bells blaring in her head. Assuming that if Pascale repeated this story to the organizers of the intercultural exchange, my name would become a dirty word, and so decided to protect us from one another.

From then on, when I called to talk to my lover, my mother told me that Pascale "*didn't want to speak to me*". It was a lie. But the motives were as I expressed. Likewise, and for the same reasons, when Pascale asked "*if I called*", and I had called repeatedly, she was told that I "*had not*". Young

Pascale was devastated, finally returning to her native Pontarlier near Switzerland, depressed and longing for her man to come rescue her.

I didn't have her address, or phone, and didn't know she was in Pontarlier, and didn't know how to reach her in France. The Internet was not yet a reality and no one had e-mail addresses, and I would have had to hire a French private detective at some ungodly cost to try to find this girl in all of France. When I divorced from Patty a few months later, I remained single for some time, trying everyone I knew to get Pascale's phone number, or some means to find her.

Three Years of Loneliness End

Likewise she waited nearly three years for her Knight to arrive on a white horse to sweep her off to New Jersey. That day never came.

Finally, alone and depressed about my loss, I began to look for feminine companionship. I was ready to start a family, and knew that my parents desperately wanted Jewish grandchildren. So, I went to a Jewish singles group and ran into Stephanie, who was the one I thought, to have my children. I was still young and foolish enough to find the idea of virginity sexy, and it fed my ego despite nagging thoughts from my "*inner voice*" that a girl who could wait until 27 in this day and age, might not have a normal libido. My inner guide was to be proven 100% right after my daughter was born. I had made another major mistake, this time, except for my children, the worst one of my life. I was simply a means to get inseminated and supported.

Another Mistake

Soon I was married to Stephanie. Did I love her when I married her? I really wanted to. And, I am sure that I never gave her even the slightest reason to think otherwise. Then, one afternoon, I was walking near the house, and ran into an old friend who had been involved in the exchange program which brought Pascale to me. During the conversation, she said *"I was talking to Pascale the other day, and she asked me to give you her number. Apparently she would like to hear from you"*. My heart sank to my stomach. What had I done? Oh dear God, what to do? I went home and cried, and though I am not religious, I prayed for some advice, because the weight of my situation was too much to bear alone, and yet I had to carry this myself. Certainly I couldn't ask Stephanie.

Regardless, I called Pascale. Coincidentally Stephanie and I were preparing a trip to Europe , a belated Honeymoon, and while there, Stephanie suggested that we *"visit"* my *"old friend Pascale"*. Naturally she had no idea that I was still desperately in love with her. But, one must realize that at this point I didn't know that Pascale was in love with me as well. After all I had not seen her for several years.

The Encounter

The day arrived that we found ourselves in Lausanne, Switzerland, a stones throw from Pontarlier, and, believe it or not, at Stephanie's urging, I called Pascale, who instantly accepted the suggestion that we come over. This was Stephanie's biggest mistake..... and I too, should have known better. For once Pascale and I could see one another's eyes.... I knew. Oh God, I knew.... The sadness I saw there because we were not alone and could not embrace, was something which I thought, would haunt my soul to the day I died. Still, I could not show my pain to my new wife. But in that instant, I knew that Pascale loved me still, and I had made another and now critical mistake in re-marrying too soon. What to do?

Soon after returning home to the States, I found out that Stephanie was pregnant with my son Bobby. And, though a part of my soul was still in Pontarlier, I had certainly "*made my bed*" now, and I determined to make the most of it and be good to Stephanie.

It needs to be said here, that Pascale and I agreed that neither she nor I would turn back the clock, if it meant that our Children had never been born, because for the most part they made all the sacrifices worth it.

Pascale Returns

Pascale, on the other hand, had other ideas. She was apparently not going to give up on me so easily. She saved her money, and soon called me to announce that she was coming to New Jersey. She had arranged to room at the home of some Native American guy she found in Palisade Park, who was only too happy to have her come here. She, on the other hand was uninterested in him, but needed the host to be able to afford the stay here. Anyway she expected to spend her time at the Press' home. When she arrived here, she was by now 21, and had gone from a cute, sweet, child of 18, still carrying a little "*baby fat*", to one of the most exquisite women I had ever seen. She was I thought then, everything I had ever dreamed of in a woman. Absolutely stunning. And still her eyes cried out for me... soon I would hear the words too.

By now Stephanie was about eight months pregnant, and not always in the best of sorts to play hostess to our friend. Trusting me completely, one evening she told me "*Stephen, I don't feel well. Take Pascale out to dinner, and show her the area*". We left together, and for the first time were able to talk freely without my wife's omnipresence.

Why Am I Not Your Wife?

Over dinner, she looked at me.... tears in her eyes, and said "*Stephen, why am I not your wife? All I EVER wanted for my life was to be Mrs. Press."* My eyes soaked over and I replied.... "*what am I to do? You know why... You know what happened. I can't leave her like this. I have to be able to sleep at night, and I would be a monster if I could do such a thing*". We went somewhere to just sit together for a few hours and we mostly just cried together.

Shortly afterwards, Pascale returned to Pontarlier. Realizing that her love was now unavailable to her, and, on the rebound, married a guy who was a willing suitor. She and Didier started a family. When my son was born, we gave him a name which was equally viable in English and in French, Robert Michael... my daughter too, Alyssa Nicole. When Pascale's first born came along, he was called Kevin, her others were also given names which were as American as French; Jordan and Timothy. And not without an ulterior motive. Somewhere in the back of both of our minds was the thought that someday we would be together.

"Maybe Someday When We Are Old"

Keeping all of this to myself was a huge strain, but I never communicated a whisper of my feelings about her to Stephanie. During those first years with her, our relations were ok, and despite my pain, together we befriended Pascale and Didier, who came back here and stayed with us. Whenever Pascale and I saw each other though, the eyes told us that we still loved one another, and there was great sadness, though simultaneously great joy at just being in the same room.

Discarded Like An Old Shoe

After some seven years, and a couple of years after my daughter was born, Stephanie came to completely reject me physically, and I was left to contemplate a life of utter celibacy, or to find an extramarital outlet. Not being one to ever cheat, I confronted her on numerous occasions, and begged her to "*get help, medical, psychological or counseling*". She would have none of that, telling me that this was "*how God made her*", that she had "*no need for intimacy*" with me, and "*didn't want to change anything*". I explained that I was "*too young to remain celibate the rest of my life, and"* if she *"would not get help, then I would start to look around*". At this, she told me… "*If I find you've been with another woman, I'll leave you*"…. I asked her if she "*thought it was fair to demand to eat her cake and have it too?*" … she just glared at me. Obviously she assumed that I should just remain celibate forever.

When I ultimately told her I had to start looking around, she told me that I was "*old and ugly…. Go see who will have you*". So, I did! It so happened that business then, due to the unique situation of the break-up of the Soviet Union, took me regularly to Moscow. There I found there were a lot of beautiful young women who were only too happy to meet an American doctor. Knowing that Pascale was now married and had already had two children, I met and foolishly married Tanya, my 4th wife, and 3rd mistake…. Parenthetically, that inner voice was screaming at me not to marry her, because I didn't really trust her, and I felt her very inconsiderate, but as some pundit said, God seems to have given men a head and a penis and only enough blood to run one at a time. Unfortunately, once again I listened to the *sotto voce* instead of the *voce interiore.*

Later, I would hear that Stephanie went to my Brother's ex-wife, who was his ex because he caught her in an extramarital affair with a Colleague of mine. So, Stephanie naturally jumped to the assumption that Carol was a expert in sexual matters. Carol told my mother that Stephanie asked her…. "*Carol, you're an experienced woman…*" the implication already something that Carol didn't like…. But she went on anyway… "*after the children are born, how long does a man expect a woman to "do her wifely duty"*?" Carol was dumbstruck! I'm told her answer was…

"*well, as far as I understand, until the day he dies, and maybe especially on that day*"! It was clearly not what she wanted to hear.

All the time, due to the lack of communications with Pascale, I didn't know she was unhappy. After all, Pascale thought I was happy, and thanks to a semblance of a French Catholic ethic, wasn't going to undermine what she thought was a good relationship with Stephanie to tell me she was miserable. I later learned that when she heard I re-married Tanya (who in retrospect was a Pascale look-alike, of sorts)… she became more depressed and because of this, determined to really try to make things work with Didier, so they had yet another child.

Wife 4, Mistake # 3

We were not together very long in the States, when I realized that I was making a huge mistake marrying Tanya. Before she came here, I had taken an admittedly small apartment around the corner from my house so we could live together, while I finalized the divorce with Stephanie.

Exile

It was supposed to be a very short exile from my home. Stephanie, ever the conniver, and I were, thought I, trying to do this on an amicable basis. Little did I realize that behind the scenes she was planning to do me dirt. One afternoon she approaches me and innocently asks, "*Stephen, the children were born here… maybe you would agree to move out for just a couple of months, until they get used to the idea of our splitting up, so they won't feel, like you're throwing them out of their home?*" Stupidly, I fell for it. It would be nearly three years before I got my house back. And, she had free run of my office at night, while I couldn't even get an Order to keep her parents from rummaging through my files. I therefore was forced to bring all my financial records into my private office every night before I could leave.

Despite the ruse to get me out of the house, and my anger about it, I tried desperately to maintain an amicable relationship with Stephanie, "*for the sake of the kids*", if for no other reason. As soon as we determined at the *pendente lite* hearing the amount of my support, I provided well for them all. In fact, whenever I left town on travel, I handed her an extra thousand dollars in cash, for emergencies. She always returned it intact, so I tried to keep trusting her. I knew she needed work then, so I gave her the option to keep on collecting the Accounts receivable for the practice she had been doing for some time, offering to pay her. I forgot that she had been made signatory to the company checking account, and when I was finally forced because that was what her lawyer demanded in the final settlement, to pay support through the probation department's support office, I tried to pay by company check. The idiotic bureaucracy kept returning my checks, claiming that they could accept a company check, but not a personal one, but couldn't accept them with my signature on them. Since I WAS the company, then who was to sign the checks?

It seemed quite mad. I was trying to pay. The money was there to pay her, but the Probation department preferred to send back my checks uncashed rather than take a valid, covered check with my signature. Madness!

Finally, after Stephanie, through the stupidity of the system hadn't received a check for about six or eight weeks, I went to the bank to get a certified check to pay them. After making out the check, and having the branch manager go to prepare it for me, she comes back to inform me that there are "*no funds in my account.*" When I inquire in my angst, what happened to my money? I was told that Stephanie had come in a few days before and cashed a counter check and drained the account. Naturally, I took her name off the signature card immediately, and fired her from the collection job.

Still that wasn't enough for Stephanie. She has the probation department come after me, and we are in Court the following Friday morning. In the meantime, she gets my son, who must have been all of six at the time to come to me crying, "*daddy... mommy says we need to buy food, and she needs you to pay the support money*". I was forced to explain that "*mommy had just drained all the money out of my account behind my back and now wanted it twice*". Imagine? How could a mother use her child like that?

Crime Pays

In Court on Friday, her lawyer tried to get the Court to Order the freezing of a corporate account , of funds which were not mine, but that of the partners in the Moscow clinic. I was being paid a salary from these funds, but had they been frozen, the partners would have sued me to get their money and I would have been cut off from those funds, thus lowering any chances of my paying her what she wanted. Despite her theft, the Family Court still Ordered me to pay the child support a second time! Who says crime doesn't pay?

If it seems like I am going back and forth between the wives, it's only because that's how it was happening... I was between the two of them all the time. Scylla and Charibdis.

I would come home to Tanya after working at my home/office and she would nag me to just give Stephanie the house, and start over... in Russia! Then she'd have fits of anxiety about our "*living like homeless people*". Next, she'd run off about the apartment being too small, so we couldn't have friends over. Etc. etc., etc.... no end in sight. Clearly if I wanted to sleep with Tanya, I would have to keep my problems entirely to myself. One night, it got so bad I actually drove to Bergen Pines, and strongly suggested that she check herself in.

So, why did I marry her after all that? Two real reasons; first, I had brought Yura here, and allowed his father to give him up so he could have a life in the US. And, I already loved him as my own son. And, second; I had given my word. The price for this honesty would be far more than I could ever imagine then.

The problems continued with Tanya unceasingly. One day we drove to Barnes and Noble's in Paramus, and as I pulled into the parking lot, an SUV pulled into the space next to us. Tanya leaned out across my lap, and started barking at the family, wildly, like a rabid dog. "Rufffff, rufffffff.... Grrrrrr".... So convincingly, that the poor guy grabbed his family and pushed them back into the van and sped off, presumably scared to death she might bite them. I too left, too mortified to get out of the car. But I stopped at a Grand Union store on the way home and came out with a small package, which I gave to Tanya. I had bought her a rawhide bone. They didn't sell muzzles! Telling her, if you ever get the urge to bark again, just chew on this instead. She thought the whole affair a riot. I was fuming.

On numerous occasions, we would be entertaining friends from Europe, driving them around New York City... and as we'd pass a nice building, Tanya would announce... "*one day when Stephen dies, I'm going to use his life insurance to buy a flat in that building*" !!

Or, she'd just tell me straight out that one day, "*I'll leave you for a younger man*". I told her there were "*no chains, go now!*"

I finally had enough, and so by 1997, I told her I wanted out. This one I would leave. The other left me. She threatened me, saying "*I'll keep you so busy answering phony accusations, with the licensing board, the IRS, the FBI, the CIA, and whoever else will hear me that your parents will be lucky if they don't have to sell their home to save you.*". Naively I inquired, "*why would you lie to the authorities, when I haven't done anything wrong?*". She said with an intense glare filled with hatred, "*no one leaves me*".

Frankly, I was a tad terrorized. I needed my practice to support my children, and I feared that she would raise such a stink, albeit phony, that it would hurt my ability to earn a living. I really had no desire to deal with this kind of wrath, and figured that such rancor would show itself in some other form if I let things die down. So, I bided my time. Waited for her to make a mistake. A couple of weeks later, after we were not really talking for a while, she came to me apologetic, saying "*let's make up... I really didn't mean all that... I wouldn't really do such things*". I responded, "*ok, if you write down that you threatened me with phony charges, and that it was all a lie, that there is nothing to charge me with.... In other words, finally tell the truth*". She did. I kept that letter in my safe. I knew that I would need it one day.

That day came in 2002, when I became friendly with Robert Maurice James Paul Alexander, His Excellency, the Count Von Glück und Kuefstein. We met one evening at the skating rink. Robert was gay, and very obviously so. I had long had cordial relationships, i.e., was on friendly terms with various gay men, as I was a skater, and also have gay relatives. I support their right to civil rights and fair treatment completely.

I'm a Lesbian

Robert, as I knew him then, was a brilliant Homeopathic Physician, and equally talented linguist, and skated at the gold level too. We obviously had much in common, and at the end of the evening, a couple of guys were going out for a burger and cup of coffee, so I invited Robert to come along with us. He said with a swish, "*you know, I'm Gay*?". I answered without batting an eyelash, "*well, so am I……… but I'm a lesbian*"…. He practically rolled on the floor… apparently no straight guy had ever said that to him before.

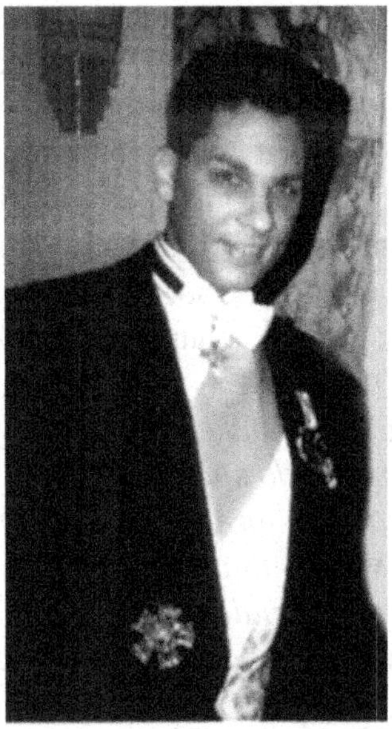

Fig. 7 H.E., the Count Von Glück und Kuefstein

In the months that followed, Robert would become perhaps my best friend. He is a complicated guy with lots of personal issues. When he had money, (now he's a Buddhist Priest sworn to poverty) he was generous to a fault; inviting me out several evenings a week to get me away from Tanya… for my own good. In the beginning, he tried to be nice to her. But it was to no avail. No matter that he invited Tanya and I, Yuri (Tanya's son) and Ruth Warrick, the actress, to the Carlisle Hotel for Thanksgiving Dinner. She refused to believe that he is a Count, convinced that he's a male prostitute, gigolo, or something dishonest, her constant disparagement of my friend made my life even more of a

Hell than before. Still I refused to discard a friend just because she had these vile ideas. Forgetting for the moment that he had just sent me around 16 patients, and that alone should have been reason enough for her to be nice to him, or at least tolerate his presence in our lives.

Robert knew that it was causing more trouble, and really tried again to be nice to her despite it. One evening we were in the City, having dinner with a classmate of hers at the Cajun restaurant on 8th Ave. She asked Robert, "*what do you do for a living*?" His Excellency retorted... "*work?, I don't work*!". "*No one in my family has ever worked*".

Then she crossed the final frontier. She said... "*so then you're a parasite*!". After that, the referrals stopped, and he never suggested she come along to dinner again. But, I had had it. Even forgetting our friendship, if she could insult someone who was feeding us with patients, she had to go, at any cost. She would surely destroy my career, my credibility and my ability to support my family.

It was soon after this that I told her for the last time, "*It's over*". I left her. Not for Robert, like she insinuated to my parents, or for Pascale for that matter. I just left Tanya out of self preservation.

The Producers

At one point, Robert was still trying to help Ruth Warrick, and myself at the same time. One afternoon at Ruth's apartment, he decided to take us both to see "*The Producers*" while it still had the original cast. He got only balcony seats, and there was no elevator. This was a problem, because Ruth had just left a nursing home after breaking her hip, so we had to form a carry with our arms and we literally lifted this Grand dame of the stage, screen and tv to balcony seats. As if this were not funny enough, as we were climbing the stairs. Robert sees an old friend and calls out "Arlene !"... It was Arlene Dahl, and her young husband. Arlene comes over seeing Ruth being carried like she had been in her movies and comments.. "where did you get the Nubians?".

Blissfully unaware of the plot, I sat between Ruth who needed a walker to get around and Robert the gay Austrian Count. Watching the number with the little old ladies with walkers, she seemed jealous that she hadn't thought to try out for the part.... And then the Gay German-Nazi numbers... I tried, but couldn't stifle my laughter.... It was hysterically funny, but I was afraid to laugh for fear I would offend someone to my right OR to my left.

It Just Goes On And On

Meanwhile, where Pascale was concerned, it would not be until Didier became really abusive that Pascale determined to get out. However the crazy laws in France at that time, made it extremely dangerous financially, for a woman with children to just walk out of the marital home, and so, she stayed and planned her escape. Their system provided that she could lose her children to him, if she did this, and would receive not a *sous*.

During this whole period, we had been in periodic phone communications, during which our pre-arranged code for "*I still love you*" was "*everything remains the same*", a parting expression we emotionally exchanged in every call.

She Disappears

Suddenly about 1997, I was unable to call her, and didn't have a clue why. Ideas ran rampant like mice running around in my brain, that maybe she no longer wanted to hear from me, or worse. It turns out that Didier came to believe that she was cheating on him, and had their phone placed on the "*red list*" (this is an unlisted phone service , but supposedly much more strictly secured than here). In reality she was never unfaithful to him, but was working part-time during school hours to develop a career of her own, so she could regain some independence to allow her eventual escape of his abuse.

It was to be some three or four years before I heard from her again. By the sheerest of serendipity, it was only two weeks after I finally told Tanya I'd had enough, that I received a postcard from Pascale, saying "*I left him, I'm alone, if you still love me, call*". I got on the phone immediately and we began making plans to meet. This just coincided with my telling Tanya it was over, by two weeks. Imagine! Just about two weeks after I actually leave Tanya, I get the note from Pascale! Wow! Parenthetically, naturally, Tanya blames not herself and her horrendous treatment of me, but Pascale. Pascale, whom I had not spoken to for some years was suddenly Tanya's scapegoat. Same way, I guess that Stephanie blamed Tanya for "*Stealing me*" from her. Strange what rationalizations go on in women's minds when they discard their men, and the guy has the nerve to leave....

Finally, We Are Both Free!

At the time I was Vice-Chairman of the Medical Commission for FIDE, the World Chess Federation, and the World Rapid Chess Championships were coming up in Cannes, on the French Riviera. I would be alone in Cannes, in the Summer, at a palace class hotel, all prepaid and courtesy of FIDE. I asked if Pascale could get away to meet me, and she jumped at the chance.

I asked if she was "*ready to stay in a hotel room with a man she had not seen in 17 years*", and her answer "*oh yeah*!" confirmed my fantasy, and that our desire was still mutual...... Then she asked me if "*I was sure that I would still find her attractive after all this time?*" I told her that it was she I loved "*and not her body*" but that privately, I felt I knew her well enough to say this, because I could be reasonably sure that she had kept herself up well, and would not disappoint me. After all I told her, "*I had always believed that to know what a girl would look like after 20 years, one should look at her mom*", and "*I remembered that her mother was an attractive lady when we were in France*"...at an age approximately equal to Pascale's now. She just laughed, and told me she would "*send me a photo so I could make sure before making a commitment*".

The Cake Has Great Icing

Finally, I said that "*if she were still beautiful, it would just be icing on the cake*". Her photo arrived and I nearly fell over... Pascale was even more devastatingly gorgeous then when I last saw her! I had to be the luckiest man on Earth!... I thought. When I called her she asked me what I "*thought of the photo*"? I replied that "*this cake has exquisite icing*"!

Seventeen Years of Exile End

Finally, the time to depart for Cannes came. It was not without incident, as Tanya decided despite that we had already agreed that we could each see others, that I should have trouble. She confronted me, saying "*you think you're going to France?.... ha! You're going to jail instead.*" I asked "*what did I do to warrant going to jail?*" She said, "*it doesn't matter, my lawyer told me that all I have to do is tell the Police that you touched me and they'll arrest you*". I said, "*but I haven't touched you*". She laughed. Luckily Yura was present all the time. He came in and said, "*mom, why would you lie to the Police? I won't let you hurt dad like that.... I'll tell them what you're doing*". She would exact revenge on him for being honest too. Yura was soon unceremoniously shipped to Moscow, to stay with relatives until the divorce ended and I could rescue him.

The next morning I flew into the nearby town of Nice. I sat around the airport for two hours, which just seemed like 2 weeks, to await my love's arrival... after all, remember, I had not seen her in 17 long years. My vision of loveliness glided down the runway, running into my arms, and we sailed over to the hotel in a taxicab, perhaps the longest half hour ride of my life. Something right out of Hollywood.

It would turn out however, that fantasy was better than reality. I hate smoking, and she was now a serious smoker. That had to stop, and she seemed willing to quit for me, but warned that it would "*ruin her mood*"... that it did! After a pretty short romantic interlude for such a long separation from one's "*true love*", she was incredibly eager to run out and shop. Then there was the list of goals with which she presented me. After a Mont Blanc pen and Louis Vuitton pocketbook, I was third on her list.... Another possession to acquire!

Still, with such an investment in this relationship, and since she was such an incredibly gorgeous lady, I was willing (again) to accept some problems, so I invited her to the States, and she came during some of the worst times I was experiencing with Tanya in our divorce. Robert, meanwhile, was telling me that his "*spirit guides*" informed that I was making a huge mistake. Little did I realize...

Rejection

One afternoon, I had to run to Court for something with Tanya, and came back in about one hour. I was feeling really depressed, and asked my lover for a hug. She looked at me and just said "*no*". She wasn't joking, she meant no! I asked if it "*was a joke*?" And she told me she "*simply was not in the mood to hug me*". I lost it, and nearly sent her to the airport then and there. But it was really an incident at the hotel in Cannes that determined that I had lost my ardor for a future with her. One evening we were talking, and without being prompted, she related an incident at another resort when "*some Arab guy who owned a hotel there and was incredibly rich*", became "*fixated*" upon her. She told me that he gave up his business and left his family to come to ask for her hand. She insisted that she had done nothing to encourage him, but it certainly seemed a very odd behavior for a serious businessman with no encouragement at all….. still it was not the story, but the smile on her face as she told it that scared me. I awoke that night in a cold sweat, having dreamed that I was with a lady whose sadistic specialty was the destruction of men's lives… a sort of sexual black widow, if you will. Of course this was just a nightmare, wasn't it? …. It wasn't the story she told, but her apparent glee at the result that made me wince.

Still, I wasn't ready to call this quits.

Goodbye

Reflecting constantly on Pascale's behavior, during our last encounter in New York and on some subsequent discussions, I was forced to think that a normal reaction to her Arab guy story, if there were really no encouragement to this kind of falling on a sword for her, would have been at least pity, embarrassment, and sadness that she should have been the cause of such self-destructive folly. I still can't say that this was Pascale, but my "*inner voice*" was screaming at me to get out. And, one must understand that I had paid too dear a price in the past for failing to heed my inner voice.

I wrote her a goodbye letter. One of the most painful things I have ever done in my life.

The silver lining in that cloud was that finally I was over the Pascale virus which had infected me for the previous twenty years. That nightmare in Cannes; was it about my life? About my marriages? I may never be able to answer that for sure, but I was now free of the infection. Did I love her still ? No. Would I always care about her? Of course.

The Next Nightmare

The story does not end there. After about two years of singleness, and dating other women, I received a letter from Pascale, telling me a very, very sad, story.

After she returned to France from her trip here, she went to Spain with her parents and children. Upon her return, she was told at work that they had retained a new accountant, and that she would be working with him. A family man of 52, two children, and a grandchild, this ugly man was quite overweight at 110 kilos. At first the association was professional, though she relates that there was "*something she found scary about him*", and couldn't tell exactly what.

The Howling

Later, she relates, "*he began to howl all the time*" making it difficult to concentrate on her work, and told her "*he wanted her*", an offer she refused in the clearest of terms.

This failed to stop his fixation upon her, and she tells that he began to stalk her, following her everywhere, calling her at her private phone number and harassing her at all hours. He then told her that he was connected with the French authorities and had high-level influential friends in the French Police and that if she reported him, no one would do anything to protect her. He told her that if she did not submit, "*soon there would be three orphans*", and he would kill her parents as well as her children and her. He showed her a bullet, and told her that the gun was "*in the car, waiting to do my bidding*".

Rape and Sodomy

She changed her phone to the red list again, and again but he would call nearly the next day! It appeared for all the world like he indeed had high level friends who could obtain such secure information from France Telecom. She was understandably terrorized and as a mother would, trying to protect her children with no authorities to help, put her body between the danger and her brood. She began to submit to a series of rapes, sodomy and other atrocities which left her nearly catatonic, when at one point she seriously contemplated suicide. Thank God she at the last second told her psychiatrist and he called the Police and this monster was arrested. When her letter came, it bore the return address of a Psychiatric hospital near her home.

She told me what occurred and that she needed my friendship. Would I still be her friend? I called immediately, and found that by the time I received the missive she had been checked out of the hospital by her dad, and was in Pontarlier with her children and her folks.

She awaits the outcome of the French legal system, and hopefully this cretin will receive his just desserts.... But fears are rampant, as just in time for this monster, the French government changed their Napoleonic Code to allow for "*presumption of innocence*" and he is out on bail! So, he returns to work, and it is Pascale who remains in a kind of arrest due to her psychological hell...placed there by this rapist monster.

For her, however, there is a ray of sunshine. Eventually this monster was found mentally incompetent to stand trial, and confined indefinitely to a hospital for the criminally insane. Since then, Pascale summoned the inner strength to kick her pills and force herself to work on getting her life back. I have full confidence in her ability to do just that.

Chapter 5

Chiropractic Enters the Olympic Games

**

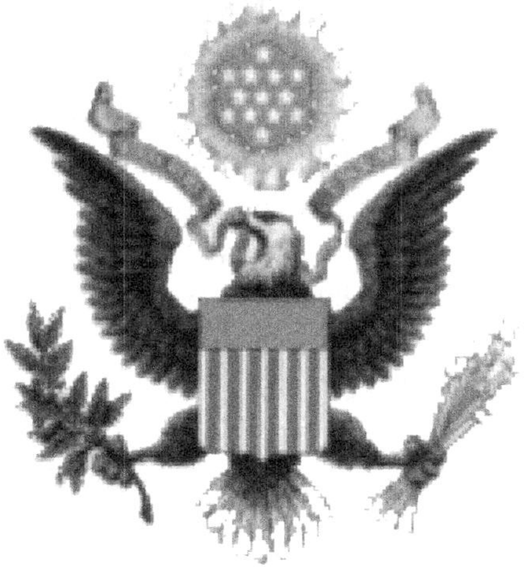

It was the beginning of my career in Chiropractic, around 1978, when I graduated from Palmer College, in Davenport, Iowa.

Developing a practice was really difficult in those days, as you might imagine, with a total prohibition against direct mail advertising, and only the most plain, professional advertisements allowed in newspapers, and the yellow pages. No display ads, nothing.

A Run at Politics

So, I decided to run for office in my town. An opening came up to run for Councilman-at-large on the Republican ticket. No one can win city-wide election as a Republican in Englewood, because of demographics. But it gave me the opportunity to walk door to door with community leaders and be introduced to every resident in the community. I became known overnight.

Shortly after opening up I joined the then fledgling ACA[4] Sports Council. The venerable Leonard Schroeder, DC, of Oak Park, Illinois, was the Founder of the Council, which formed about 1977. At that time, there were perhaps 25 or 30 active members nationwide. At that time none of the health professions had a board certification in Sports Medicine, and the whole specialty was in its infancy.

A Great DC is Martyred

At the same time, a pioneer in sports Chiropractic, Leroy Perry, DC of California, had already managed to be a team doctor in the Olympic Games. In those days, since there was no Internationally accepted protocol for "*finagling*" these appointments, one could approach a third-world Nation's Olympic Committee, and by providing "*financial incentives*", errr… a donation, one could get oneself

[4] American Chiropractic Association

appointed. Naturally there is no proof of the means by which Dr. Perry got himself into "*the Games*", but suffice it to say, he was there as early as the 1976 Games in Montreal. I believe he was representing Aruba as their team Doctor.

The import to the future of our profession of this seemingly small initial incursion cannot be overestimated, because all of the efforts of all those who came later, would have taken much longer to accomplish what has come since without his single-mindedness and foresight. The athletes apparently loved him, and he brilliantly ingratiated himself with not only the US and the Aruban team, but the US Athletes themselves, and, in some ways more importantly the Cubans. The great boxer Alberto Juantarena, known to his fans as "*El Cavallo*" was an immediate devotee.

A couple of years prior to the 1980 Winter Olympic Games taking place in Lake Placid, NY, Dr. Perry was positioning himself to achieve his goal of being the first US Olympic Team DC. He had befriended, and treated many important athletes, like Dwight Stones, the Gold medal high jumper, and sometime in 1979 appeared on National Television, on Tom Snyder's "*Tomorrow Show*" together with Dwight Stones.

During the interview, which did wonders for sports Chiropractors nationally, Dwight Stones made an otherwise innocent comment which would prove to be the undoing of Dr. Perry's goal. He said "*I would not have won my medal if not for Dr. Perry*". Taken in today's context, one could not conceive of a reason that would be anything but taken as high praise. But in 1979 the attitude of the USOC under the Kane administration, shortly after the IOC tenure of the infamous Avery Brundage, was still "*then why have Dwight Stones jump at all? Just give the medal to Dr. Perry*".... sarcasm of course, but reflective of their thinking. The result of this brouhaha was that, Dr. Perry, a hero pioneer to those of us in sports Chiropractic, became so anathema to the

USOC that Olympically anyway he was martyred to the cause of Sports Chiropractors everywhere.

Happy Happenstance Brings a Juxtaposition

In that context then understand that I was practicing in Englewood, NJ. The same town as Irving Dardik, MD, a renowned vascular surgeon, who was serendipitously serving as Chairman of the USOC Sports Medicine Commission, since, as I understand, he was a friend and physician to Mr. Jack Kelly, President of the USOC, who in a cruel twist of fate, dropped dead while running and motivated Dardik to devote his life to finding the cause.

Dr. Schroeder and his board of directors, were actively engaged in the pursuit of information about the members of the USOC Sports Medicine Commission, and up to that point, had not been given the time of day by the USOC administration.

All this information is background to the fact that at just that time, at the end of my first year in practice, I received a letter from Dr. Schroeder addressed to: "*All members of the ACA Sports Council*", asking if anyone "*knew any of the names of the USOC Sports Medicine Commission?*"

The next week, again coincidentally, I found myself invited by the East Bergen Ambulance Association, to videotape a disaster drill being held at Englewood Hospital. In yet another happy coincidence, I had purchased early video equipment, to develop a research project I was running involving gait biomechanics in skaters. Thus I was one of the few people in the area with such sophisticated gear, and was in demand for such events. At Englewood Hospital, while standing in the Emergency Room, where I was the video guy, not acting as a DC.... I found myself standing next to the partner of Dr. Dardik, Dr. Ibrahim Ibrahim, whom I engaged in conversation.

During the course of that conversation, I mentioned the letter from Dr. Schroeder, and the fact that the ACA was trying to accomplish a rapprochement with the USOC, and inquired whether Dr. Ibrahim thought that the illustrious Dr. Dardik would deign to meet with the likes of us? He told that he saw no reason why not, and invited me to call to their offices on Monday next. Naturally, I did exactly that, and quickly found myself talking to Dr. Dardik.

He mentioned that he "*was under some pressure to find a solution to the athlete's demands for a DC in the team*", and thought that maybe if we entered into a dialogue we could arrive at some solution. It was agreed to arrange a meeting, and I immediately called the very surprised Dr. Schroeder, who till then had never heard my name. I asked him "*would you like to meet the Chairman of the Olympic Sports Medicine Commission?*", and was somewhat shocked to hear his ask me "*who is it*?" After assurances that this was not a bad joke, but for real, he told me he'd "*call me right back*".

Minutes later, I got a conference call from Dr. Schroeder with the then Chairman of the ACA Board of Governors, Ralph Guenther, DC, also on the line. It was arranged that Dr. Schroeder would fly in whenever convenient to Dr. Dardik to have that meeting. I called Dardik back, and a meeting was set for the following week in the cafeteria of Englewood Hospital.

At that now historic meeting, the three of us sat down and discussed the issues regarding what the USOC thought about the "*Perry matter*". This was alluding to the fact that a member of the US Olympic Judo team, now a DC, Dr. Jim Wooley, appeared to organize a rally in Texas with the "*US Olympians Organization*", demanding a DC to work with the team. It was assumed that Dr. Perry had underwritten that event financially, and Dr. Dardik hinted that the USOC ascribed base motives to that effort.

But we were "*coming in the front door*", and according to Dr. Dardik "*doing this the right way*", and thus professionally acceptable to them. Naturally, had it not been for the pressure brought to bear by Lee Perry, and Jim Wooley and the US Olympians, our efforts would certainly have fallen on deaf ears.

An agreement was reached that Dr. Dardik, who was heading towards Colorado Springs for a meeting, would stop in Illinois, and meet with our legendary Dr. Joseph Janse at National College for a tour of one of our most prestigious institutions.

Dr. Dardik told us later that after seeing National's facilities, and talking to Dr. Janse, he went back to the US Olympic Training Center, and recommended to a sub-committee of the Commission that "*a DC be included in the Games*". He even went so far as to relate that when it came to the full Commission, a DO named Murray Goldstein who was with NIH in Bethesda, MD, asked "*why he felt he needed a DC, when DO's can manipulate*?". Dardik told us later that he simply asked Dr. Goldstein "*how many hours of Manipulation had he studied in his course at Osteopathic College?*", and when told "*about 120*", just said, "*thanks Dr., I think we'll leave it up to those who are really expert in Manipulation to adjust our athletes*".

Press Turns Down the Appointment

Dardik returned to New Jersey and promptly called my office, and asked me if I wanted to go to Lake Placid. What I answered would haunt me for the rest of my professional life, due to circumstances I could not then have foreseen. But I chose the altruistic tack, and demurred, saying "*you know I would give anything to be the first US Olympic DC, but I am in practice (then) only one year. I think it's unfair to the athletes to do this, when I know that they really want Dr. Perry*". Dardik then said, "*you know that we will NEVER [emphasis his] accept Perry*". I said, "*ok then, his work is mostly based on the work of another very well known DC; George Goodheart, in Detroit, let's ask him*".

Dardik thanked me, and as far as I knew called Dr. Goodheart himself. It turns out that this was not exactly the case either. Things now took a strange turn to cause Goodheart to believe that another DC had recommended him.

At the same time we were meeting with Dr. Dardik, a class was in session, held under the auspices of National College, at Newark Airport. It was the first [5]CCSP course, then called CTP (Certified Team Physician). And that weekend I naively, and excitedly, ok, I bragged a bit about, the events of the week ... someone there, was friendly with a DC then practicing in Dumont, NJ, named Leo Minsky. Leo was a "*Fellow*" in the [6]ICAK, Dr. Goodheart's personal, and by all other standards unaccredited, professional society, which promoted his development, known as "*Applied Kinesiology*", and I was only recently trained in this subject, and not so well connected.

By yet another accident, Minsky some years before had some dealing with Dardik, and promptly called him, mentioning that he was close to Goodheart. What followed, I do not exactly know, but for some reason Goodheart to this day mistakenly believes that it was Minsky who gave his name to Dardik.

A Felon Gets the Credit

One should know that Leo Minsky was not known as a particularly nice guy. He was subsequently arrested trying to hire a hit-man to kill his wife, and served some prison time

[5] Certified Chiropractic Sports Physician
[6] International College of Applied Kinesiology

for that. So, one could legitimately call his testimony in this matter into question. Of course, one only has to ask Dr. Dardik who gave him Goodheart's name, and I have no doubt he would corroborate this fact.

The Tai Babilonia and Randy Gardner Affair

The upshot of all this, is that when the Games came to pass, the DC present was not under any public scrutiny at all, but rather hidden from view completely. In a trailer marked only "*Sports Medicine Modalities*". And Dr. Goodheart was under a strict prohibition not to volunteer to treat anyone, unless they came looking for a DC.

This all resulted in some rather famous boondoggles. One which comes to mind was the situation involving Tai Babilonia and her partner Randy Gardner, whose groin pull took him out of the games. Goodheart had just treated a Canadian skier who looked for a Chiropractor and found Goodheart, with the same injury, and he went on to a gold

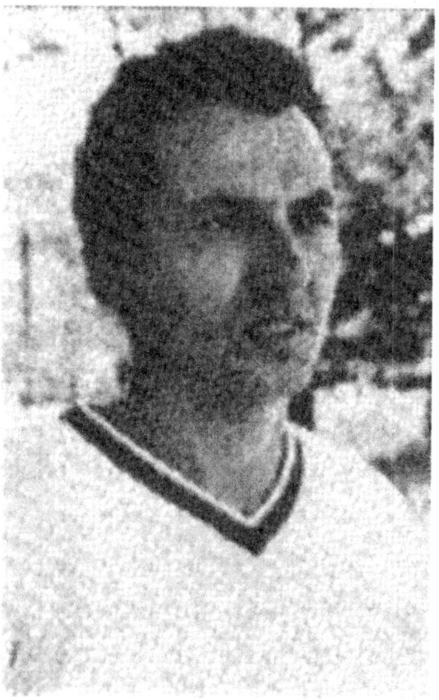

Fig 8 Irving Dardik, MD

medal. But when Randy came to the trailer to be treated by the other Docs, Goodheart kept strictly to his protocol and didn't volunteer, even privately to Dr Dardik that he could help him and Randy and his partner withdrew from the Games. Parenthetically, it seems that the sympathy this generated launched their skating careers to new heights.... So maybe it was better for Tai and Randy that George kept his mouth shut!

Shortly after the Games, Dardik called and told me that I had done the right thing. Moreover, he assured me that a program would be launched to bring DC's to the training Center to screen them for future Olympic Games. I was promised that I could be the first to go under this program. But, then Dardik lost his position at the USOC, and all that dissolved into thin air for a while.

Another Martyr to "the Cause"

Irving Dardik is a wide-eyed visionary; brilliant, talented and open-minded. The Chiropractic profession never properly thanked this man for his role in bringing Chiropractic into the Olympic movement. After the Lake Placid Games (1980), I ran into him at a US Olympic Academy held at Indiana University. He was sitting in the hall of one of their grand buildings, playing the piano like a concert master. It turns out he was self taught. "*Irv*" as he told me to call him, took enormous heat from the medical establishment for supporting us. They threatened him with loss of his malpractice insurance, and more. He ultimately lost his license to practice medicine, (today he's doing research in Calafon, New Jersey on "*heartwave therapy*") and I can't help wonder what part his support of Chiropractic played in that?

A Tragic-Comedy of Errors

An [7]ATC named Bob Beeten, and his wife Jenny Stone were in charge of the Sports Medicine program at Colorado Springs, even administratively supervising the Orthopedic surgeons who volunteered their time too. In short, if Beeten didn't like you, you didn't get to come back.

I was also attending an annual program through the USOC Education Council, called the US Olympic Academy, and willingly found myself at Colorado Springs, at the training center. A friend of mine, Dr. Sergei Aleshinsky, who at that time was a "*Visiting Professor of Biomechanics*" at the [8]OTC asked me to treat him there. We went together to ask Mr. Beeten for permission and I was summarily dismissed, permission denied. Aleshinsky later learned that Beeten had said "*that Press guy has something to do with promoting Perry*". Remember, I had never spoken to Perry, except to have had the sad duty to call him on behalf of Dardik, to tell him that Goodheart was going, not he. So, when the program Dardik promised me would happen, finally did begin some two or three years later, I optimistically filed an application, and only later learned that it was just tossed into the garbage by Mr. Beeten.

Thus lit my motivation and drive to bring other National Associations into the fold, and achieve my own Olympic aspirations.

Press becomes the first DC- Fellow

It was now about 1983, and through the kind auspices of [9]Dr. Vojin Smodlaka, and some behind the scenes help from another former Officer of the FIMS (Fédération Internationale de Medicine du Sport, the World Governing

[7] Certified Athletic Trainer
[8] Olympic Training Center
[9] Recipient of the FIMS Gold medal, and past Board member

Body for Sports Medicine) Dr. Allan Ryan[10]. I became the first, and still sole DC to be elevated to "*Fellow*" of the American College of Sports Medicine. This was a passport to acceptance into the next step in gaining the then coveted title of "*Individual Member of the FIMS*". At that time the highest credential a physician could attain in Sports medicine Internationally.

Again, being a linguist was an enormous help in this arena, as the World of sports medicine was dominated by Europeans, and they generally looked down their noses at monolingual Americans.

To become an individual member, one had to first be a Fellow of one's National body in sports medicine (I was), take and pass a FIMS Course in Sports Medicine, and then apply for membership in FIMS. Unfortunately the FIMS had never given a course in the US, nor ever in English. So, I worked on my French in anticipation of a class being planned for France later that year.

Welcome to the UK

At the last moment, a course was offered in the UK, and I arrived the day after the US bombed Libya. Naturally, the Brits were none too thrilled at having not only a DC, but a Yank DC at that !

On arrival at the Lilleshall National Sports Centre in Shropshire, I was greeted by Peter Thomas, MD, then Secretary of BASM, the British Assoc. of Sports Medicine, who told me straight off, that had I "*been a British Chiro, we would never have accepted you, but since you come from the US where Chiros are licensed and you're a Fellow of ACSM, we decided to give you a chance*".... Welcome to England!

---

[10] Past Secretary-general of the FIMS

Part-way though the class, when it became clear that I would complete the requirements, a panic apparently set in... he was to tell me directly... would they actually give me a Diploma, or not? And what if they refused?

I understand that FIMS, hearing that a DC might actually make the requirements for Individual member, (I had already applied) held an emergency meeting in Amsterdam... while I was in England. And voted to call a moratorium on individual memberships, pending their next general assembly, some three years hence! They would ultimately decide, in order to keep ME out of their ranks, that they should do away with the credential, thereby diluting its prestige for those élite Doctors who had already attained it, by "*extending Individual membership to all members of recognized National associations*", i.e. like now 14,000 "*individual members*" in the ACSM alone!

Foiled in my plans, but with the FIMS Course Diploma in my hot little hands, I went home to the US. Needless to say I was a bit steamed.

It was 1986, and just before going, the new President of the ACA Sports Council, recognizing my linguistic hobby, and the Fellow in ACSM, etc., suggested that I should serve the Council as Chairman of the International Affairs Committee, and sit on their Board as an Advisor. I gratefully accepted the appointment.

During this tenure, I was present at the Pan Am Games Scientific Congress in Indianapolis, where as Chairman of the Speaker Selection Committee for the ACA Council, I had determined to ask Dr. Lou Sportelli to fill the spot our Council had been given at the Scientific meeting.

Chiropractic Sports Medicine Journal Starts Publishing

While there, I wandered into the booth opened by Williams and Wilkins Publishing House, and casually mentioned to the lady at the counter that maybe "it was time to have a journal for Sports Chiropractic" and volunteered to help bring it together. It turned out the lady I spoke to was the W&W journals acquisitions editor, Deanna Gemmel, and she was interested indeed! So, I called Bob Hazel, who flew out on the next plane to meet with us, and "*Chiropractic Sports Medicine*" was born. Naturally, I served on their Editorial Board, until things between myself and Dr. Hazel turned ugly over the founding of FICS, and he fired me. So the only DC Fellow of the American College of Sports Medicine, the only DC to have a FIMS course diploma, and I'm no longer on the Editorial Board of the very journal that would not have existed except for any chance discussion with Williams and Wilkins. Imagine!

Dr. Hazel, in typical American "*we'll run the World*" style, asked me to write a letter suggesting that the ACA Sports Council could be an advisory body to the IOC medical commission for DC credentialing, to the IOC Medical Commission Chairman, [11]S.A., Prince Alexandre de Merode, of Belgium, whom I had met at an ACSM meeting, because another friend of mine, who was Sports Minister of the City of Buenos Aires, Argentina, Dr. Hector Adolfo "*Chacho*" Fort insisted on introducing us. I got a letter back, saying that the IOC "*recognized the good works of the ACA Sports Council*", but that we were "*just one Country*". Bye!

Thinking every night about how the World would never accept the ACA as the World Governing Body for anything. It was now clear we needed a true International Agency to represent the interests of Sport minded DC's, and went to

[11] Son Altess "His Highness"

sleep at night thinking about the FIMS and "*how to FIX those guys*"..... one morning at 4:00 AM I awoke from a sound sleep and thought.. "*FIX... FICS... Eureka*!".

I ran to my office by 4:30AM, and began making calls to Europe and the far east. I had a $4,000.00 phone bill that month but everyone loved the idea!

US Olympic Academy

It was about this time in my life that I stumbled into an old friend, Stan Wright, who was at the time, the Athletic Director of Fairleigh Dickinson University. Stan was the coach who got booted from the US Olympic Team after the black power salute in Mexico City. Naturally he had no control over that situation, but someone had to take the fall.

One day, while talking to him at his FDU office, he showed me a brochure for a then fledgling United States Olympic Academy. It was to be held at Indiana State University, in Bloomington. This was an arm of the Education Commission of the USOC, and was intended to promote the ideals of "*Olympism*" in the schools. Olympism is that set of values which are designed to inculcate sportsmanship and the idea that it is better to participate than win, better to try than not, and so on.

I went to IU, and instantly became enamored of the ideas, and returned every year for nearly eight years running. Eventually being invited to speak as "*distinguished lecturer*" at the USOA in Indianapolis one year. It was a first for me, and the first DC for them.

From hatred to a love affair

Another embarrassing story came during one of the USOA's held at SUNY Plattsburg, in upstate New York. When I was a child, I had been told not to return to several summer camps, because I hated sports! When the other kids were told we are playing ball, I refused to play, preferring to collect insects or study nature. If they forced me to take a position on the field, I usually sat down and allowed the balls to fly over my head and ignore them. It naturally infuriated everyone. So, in desperation to find somewhere I could be happy in the Summer, my folks found the Adirondack Science Camp. This was heaven for nerdy kids like I was... all the Counselors were professors at the local State College.

One day at the USOA, we were driving in a bus from the campus of SUNY Plattsburgh, to the US Olympic Training Center in Lake Placid, some 40 minutes away. I was sitting up front in the bus with Bob and Mrs. Kane (President of the USOC at the time), and with Ernie Rangazas, the Athletic Director of SUNY Plattsburgh. Engaged in conversation, Ernie asks me if I'd ever "*been in Plattsburgh before?",* and I replied, "*yes, many years ago, at a camp called Adirondack Science Camp"....* Shock overtook his face, and he blurted out.... "*You were one of MY alumni?.... but.... but.... That was a camp for kids who hated sports!!!"...* I was really mortified.... My anti-sport background exposed in front of the USOC President!!! I said.... "*yes... strange how people can change, huh???*"

Chapter 6

FICS is Founded

**

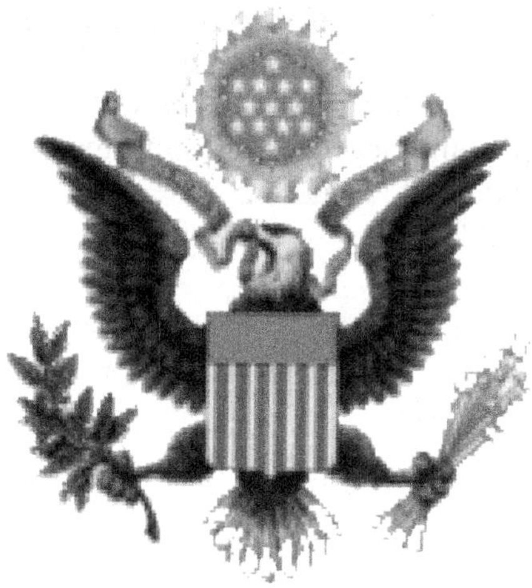

It was now early 1987. At the next American Chiropractic Association - Sports Council meeting, which was again coincidentally in New Jersey, at the Meadowlands; a conference of which I chaired the organizing committee; I suggested to the Board that we form a World Governing Body for Sports Chiropractic. Dr's Robert Hazel, Tom Hyde and John Danchik were there, as well as a few others I cannot recall at the moment.

A Plot is Foiled

I decided that we were beset by several problems at that time; a. that Chiropractors had no single agency to govern their behavior at World level meets, and this allowed some really egregious conduct at times, and it left the agency which took that DC with no one to whom to complain; and, b.-there was no credential which could be revoked. I.e. if we gave someone a Diplomate in say, sports Chiropractic, no one could take it from him/her if s/he turned out to be a real Bozo. So, I set up FICS to both provide a central registry for sports chiropractors at the World level, and also to provide two levels of membership; a-associate member, for all those DC's initially joining us, and b.-"*Full*" membership, designed to become the highest credential in sports chiropractic Internationally, for those who had distinguished themselves on International delegations, meetings service to the profession etc.... but, as a class of membership, it uniquely, could be revoked!

I was not only rebuffed, but Dr. Hazel hatched a plan to oust me from the Board, presumably for preaching the heresy that the ACA should not run the world? A friend dropped a dime on their plans, and I came back to this otherwise clandestine meeting. After all, as a Board member still, I had a right to be there. So, I decided to take the weight off them for having to throw me out without due process, and I gave them a resignation letter stipulating that the resignation was effective six months hence. This gave me another few months to organize the Fédération Internationale de

Chiropractique [sic]Sportive [12], while still legitimately representing that I was a Board Member of the ACA Council!

Someone in the UK informed that there were plans for an International Chiropractic Associations Presidential Summit, to be held in England in September 1987, and I was given the name of Dr. Arne Christiansen of Denmark, who was, I think, affiliated with the Anglo-European Chiropractic College in Bournemouth. Christiansen was in charge of the organizing committee. I promptly called Dr. Christiansen, and was given a room to meet to form the FICS.

The Charter is Signed

Among those I called to create a charter, were Drs. George Billauer of California, who had been US Team DC at the US Olympic Festival; John Stump, then of Alabama, President of the ICA[13] Sports Chiropractic Council; Jacques Bréton, President of the Canadian College of Chiropractic Sport Sciences; and Dr. Noel Patterson, a class-mate of mine at Palmer, and President of the Australian Chiropractic Association Sports Council. All signed a Charter Document to Incorporate in New Jersey, which I wrote myself, and filed with my own funds with the Secretary of State of New Jersey a few months before the meeting in London, at the beautiful Kensington Hall.

Calls then went back to the people at all the other National associations I had located, some of which no one else in the US even knew existed. One Country had only three DC's and they had one association, but two guys claimed to be

---

[12] This was the orignal idea for the spelling. It wasn't until I consulted the Canadian President, Jacques Bréton, that were told that this was not acceptable in Canada. So I suggested the alternative spelling "Chiropratique", and that is how this spelling came to exist. Now accepted by all the European Associations using French language.. previously they were using Chiropractic or Chiropractique

[13] International Chiropractor's Association (a smaller US Association than the ACA).

President. One Nation had only one DC, but he had two associations (lol).

Some 23 National Chiropractic Association Presidents attended the formative meeting of the FICS that day. Some couldn't immediately commit their Associations to membership and some could. So, presiding pro tem, I suggested that we take the approach that those who could commit to participation vote, and those who could not vote in good conscience due to political protocol reasons, recuse themselves, and remain as observers. About 18 representatives voted to form the FICS, including Dr. Hazel, who came to England to do this. I proffered that a Statutes, essentially reproducing that of the FIMS be accepted, because I suggested that this was a way to avoid a decade long battle with the IOC to accept a new Statutes… we could simply say that the format of our Federation was [14]*res judicata*, as they had already accepted the FIMS and we were a Chiropractic clone of the FIMS, thus instant recognition as to what and who we were!

This was accepted, and we were officially an agency. I then offered to hold elections. Dr. Hazel proceeded to nominate me as President, and someone else motioned to close the ballot. It was accepted, and I was elected by unanimous vote of the now voting members of the FICS.

This marked the first time the ACA and the ICA were brought together in any super-ordinate body.

It turned out that the WFC (World Federation of Chiropractic) was the result the next year of the Summit at which we officially organized. Thus the FICS is the World's first true International Agency to govern any aspect of Chiropractic.

---

[14] Legal term- already adjudicated

An American Conspiracy

In the aftermath of all this organizing, several National Associations gained licensure in their respective countries, using the FICS's participation as a springboard. Dr. Enrique Benet-Canut the foresighted, hard working pioneer in Mexico, saw the first of what would become many opportunities in his Country, and invited FICS at the London meeting to hold its next Executive Session in lovely Mexico City in 1988. The press coverage he got for that event was extraordinary, and we even had the Sports Minister of Mexico the Hon., Sr. Pascual Ortiz-Rubio, open our meeting.

It seems that Hazel had other reasons for coming to the meeting in London. Actually he apparently wanted to quash FICS by nominating me as President, and then undermine it at home. When he got back to the ACA Sports Council, he told them not to pay their dues, and they withheld their participation, hoping to cause our self destruction. Cute! However, at the time, the ACA and the ICA were in the throes of a merger negotiation, and the ACA really wanted the ICA to merge with them. There were numerous reasons, but one of them was to free the name "*International Chiropractor's Association*" to be a really International agency for Chiropractic, i.e. that would have been the name used for what is now the World Federation, but the merger ultimately failed.

When Hazel found out we were meeting in Mexico City, he cunningly convened a Board meeting for the same weekend, ostensibly to prevent any member of his Board from coming to Mexico City and giving the ACA's report. He even called me up and threatened me, saying that if anyone had the nerve to try to represent the ACA Council, he'd "*come down on me so hard, my head would spin*".

What to do? Dr. Canut, President of the Mexican Association was a Chancellor at a College here, Sherman

Straight College of Chiropractic, that was closely allied with the ICA, and which, due to the merger attempt, the ACA wanted to weaken. So, we got him to invite the Chairman of the ACA Board of Governors, Dr. Shelby Elliott, now president of Texas Chiropractic College, to the meeting. Knowing of course that due to the politics, Dr. Elliott would feel impelled to show.

FICS Wins

When he sat in on our meeting, he realized how important this really was, and asked me where the representative of the ACA Sports Council was? When I told him what was going on, he called Hazel, and ordered him to "*get his %^& to Mexico City*." He couldn't come for other reasons, so naturally it was the ACA Chairman who gave the report and Hazel didn't "*come down on me*" for that! We had won! All the important factions were included in the FICS. We were a real, International Agency representing nearly every National Chiropractic Association in the World.

Later, despite that it would not have existed but for our meeting in Mexico, Dr. Canut would conveniently never manage to name me an Honorary Member of the Mexican Sports Chiropractic Council, probably afraid it would piss off Drs. Pierson and Patterson, who seized the helm of power at FICS, forming a power clique which ran the agency for some years. All despite that the meeting in Mexico City was the basis for forming their Council and a springboard for their getting Licensing for Chiropractors in Mexico! Gratitude.... ??

The Betrayal

There would be plenty of additional intrigue to color the future of the FICS. The weight that I took on my shoulders for the enmity of those in powerful places who now had to kowtow to an association of DC's, because I thought to create FICS, would be at times hard to bear. But nothing could prepare me for the treachery of my own colleagues, some of whom would plot to bury the memory of my contribution to my profession. Even conspiring to keep me from lecturing in my own field for nearly ten years. And they actually demanded openly that I not use the title of "*Founder*" of FICS, which I, of course, founded.

In the end, truth would win over lies, and true friends and moral men, like Drs Thomas Hyde and Gordon Lawson, would restore my legacy, and see that I was finally recognized. This would come only after arranging the ouster of both the plotting Patterson and Pierson from the Board of FICS, restoring my rightful place and title, as "*Founder of the FICS*'.

Chapter 7

Algeria

**

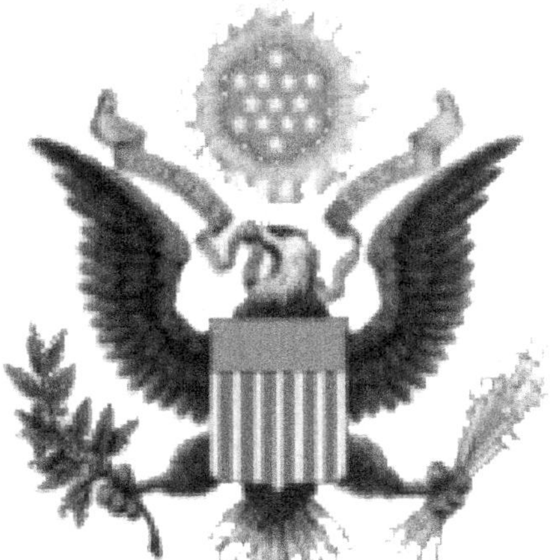

Shortly after its formation, due to the pre-FICS efforts of a couple of Sports oriented DC's, like Drs. David Pierson, then of Philadelphia, and Don Oyao of Australia; several National Olympic Committees in Africa expressed interest in having us come there to provide services at the annual African Athletics Championships, and maybe at the quadrennial African Games.

To Annaba

In 1988 the Championships were to be held in Algeria, and a group of us determined to undertake an expedition to Annaba, near the Tunisian border. As President of FICS, I notified our members that they should each obtain a Visa application from their respective Algerian Embassies, complete the requirements, and send them to me, rather than the Embassy. That way I could regulate that all were uniformly completed, and monitor the process. This was something for which I would be truly grateful later.

Knowing that we were about to embarque on what could be a dangerous journey for some of us, I sat down and wrote a manual for ethics and behavior on foreign trips, called the "*FICS Field Doctor's Guide*". It was later vetted by Pierson , and he made a couple of suggestions as to content. Later, true to form, i.e., avoid crediting Press, he claimed that the manual was a "*group effort*".

Jews Need Not Apply

In 1988, apartheid had not yet ended its ugly repression in South Africa, and I was not surprised to see a note on each application prohibiting those with South African Visas in their passports from applying. However, I was taken aback when I got the application from the Algerian Embassy in Washington, when I saw the proscription was for those with "*Visas in their passports from Israel or South Africa*"… the worst was to come, when I saw the applications from the

Algerian Embassies in other Countries, the statement was clearer… " *If you have a Visa in your passport from Israel, or South Africa, or you are a Jew do not apply*".

Great! I may not be religious, but I am Jewish, and I'm not ashamed of my heritage. But I am the Chef-de-Mission of this delegation, and can't chicken out because my ethnicity was anathema to our hosts. I called the US State Department and asked their counsel.

They told me to black out the line in the application which asks religion, and supplement nationality; US, Australian, Norwegian etc. in other words…. "its none of your business, Algeria".

We received the Work Visas anyway.

Freemasonry a crime

I arrived with the US group at Orly airport, in Paris, and was standing in line to board an Air Algerie flight to Annaba, when a flight attendant from Air France came over to me having seen my ring and asked me in French, "*are you a Mason*?". I answered "*yes, why?*". He told me that Chedli Benjidid, the then dictator of Algeria, had recently declared Freemasonry to be a capital crime. And then suggested that I check my ring in Paris. This was really nice…. A double whammy….. a Jew AND a Mason! Oh well, I hid my ring, figuring that we were going through VIP reception at Annaba, and tried to hide my nerves as well.

No VIP

Our arrival was less than VIP, but at least they didn't find my Masonic ring. So, we headed off to the "Olympic Village" to try to get someone to accept our help. It turned out only after we got there that Pierson didn't exactly have it arranged that we could work at the venue, only a vague promise that we could show up and they'd use us, from a buddy at the last annual event.... Pierson was late, and no one knew who had made the promise.

We decided to approach their officials directly. Thank God I spoke French. Initially we were told "*go home, we don't want Chiropractors here*". But when they understood that it would not cost them anything, they changed their minds. They even arranged two cars with interpreters for us; one for the group, and one for the Chef-de-Mission, me!

I stayed at the Hotel Seybouse in the center of town, the rest of the delegation stayed at the Olympic Village. The Hotel Seybouse was rated ***** , i.e., 5 stars ! When I got there, I would have given it one dirty star by our standards. It was a bit run down, un-air conditioned in the sweltering 100+ degree heat, and when we asked for ice in the restaurant, we got a tray with black stuff floating in the water with the cubes. Yuk!

Still, I had it far better than the others. I later found out that the Olympic Village didn't have hot water. There were no toilets, only holes in the ground. No Showers, only sinks. Etc., etc., etc. Not my idea of Paradise.

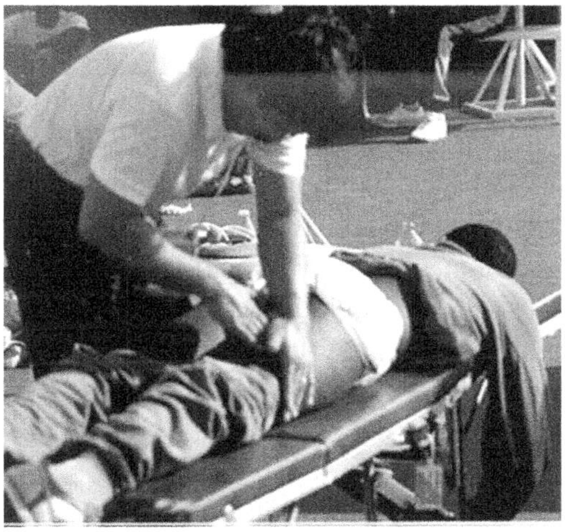

Fig 9 The Author treating an African Athlete in Annaba, Algeria

A Woman Alone

And there were constant dangers for us. Constant probing about our origins, and interesting cultural issues. One evening our group decided to go our for a French dinner, to restaurant. Off we went on foot the one and a half kilometers to the designated place. The dinner was the best meal we had had there. When we finished we started home, and stopped in a raised town square area to listen to music. There were drums like from sub-Saharan Africa, and we were entranced. We stood for some time until the lone female member of our group, Dr. Margaret Karg of Boston, turned to me and said, "*Stephen, get me out of here!*".... I asked her "*why?*" And she said "*look around you... where are the women?*" None of us guys had noticed while intent on the music, but Margaret got nervous when people started staring at her..... she was the only Female in a sea of Muslim men glaring at her!

We quietly moved out towards the hotel, and thankfully arrived in one piece, though we were all rather scared for her safety till then.

The next night, I was standing in the lobby of the Seybouse with my assigned representative of the State Protocol Committee, and in walks a delegation of Military types in uniform. I asked him, remember entirely in French, what were their ranks? (as they all had starts on their epaulets, and they seemed too young to all be Generals.

Traps

I was told "*I can't tell you that*". I asked why? He said "*you could be with the* [15]*Mossad*".

I had to think quickly….. I replied, "*If I were with the Mossad, would I have to ask you*?". Phewww….. Mossad, really!

A Hebrew Lesson

Finally, on yet another tense evening, I asked my Protocol guy on another night, "*how do you say 'Good Night' In Arabic?*". He retorted "[16]*Lila Tov*"! Of course I couldn't afford the luxury of recognition of this answer as good night in Hebrew. So what to say?

I told him, "*you know, I told you I practice near New York, which is why I am interested in foreign languages. In my office there are probably 15 different languages spoken on any given day.*" I continued, "*I had always heard that there were great similarities between Arabic and that language they speak in Israel….. Hebrew? But that sounds just like how they say Good Night"….* He replied "*yeah, that was*

[15] Israeli Secret Police
[16] Good Night in Hebrew

Hebrew". I said, "*why did you tell me that in Hebrew ? Did you want me to go out and speak to people in Hebrew? I'd get shot!*". He finished, "*no, I would have told you eventually. I just wanted see if you're an Israeli spy*". Gulp! We were surrounded by military types again and some were turning around. What to do? I said, "*YOU'RE the one who speaks Hebrew, maybe YOU'RE the Israeli spy*". He ran off, and I never saw him the rest of the trip!

The rest of the trip was uneventful except that everyone got "*Bendjidid's Revenge*" by the second day there, and we were doing a land office business in Lomotil. I was able to hold out till the eighth day… Iron stomach.!

Kissing the ground

When I got back to Kennedy Airport, my bags didn't arrive with me…. but I was so elated to be home, I actually bent down and kissed the earth!

Chapter 8

FICS to the USSR

**

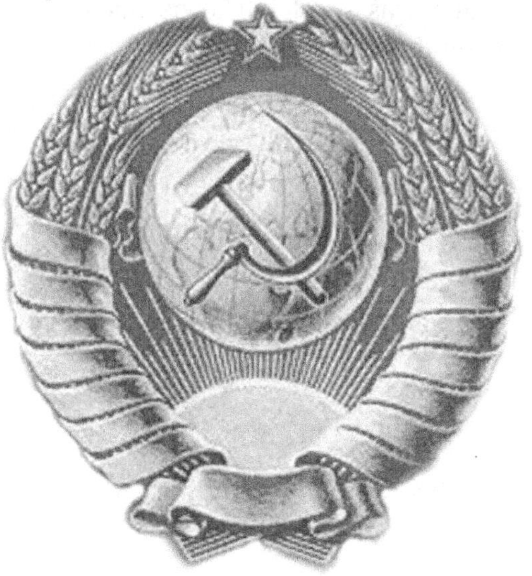

The following year after the Algeria trip, a young member of FICS, Dr. James Stoxen of Illinois, was sitting on a plane bound for somewhere, when he got into a conversation with a Dr. Edmund Enos of Montreal, Canada. Dr. Enos was an emissary to the Kremlin of the Rt Hon. Pierre Eliot Trudeau, Prime Minister of Canada. Enos had started his own agency, called the Association for Inter-Cultural Exchange Programs, or AICEP. AICEP arranged trips to Moscow and St. Petersburg etc., for sports groups to exchange views, training etc.

Dr. Stoxen's Serendipity

Jimmy Stoxen, never to miss an opportunity, talked about the possibility of FICS arranging a trip to study Sports Medicine at their National Institute of Physical Culture in Moscow. Enos was interested and made some preliminary arrangements.

I was invited to come along on a free ticket, "*if FICS got enough of a response*". Well twenty DC's from around the planet wanted in. They registered to come from Australia, Noel Patterson; Norway, Øystein Ogre; Denmark, Joseph Shafer, et al.

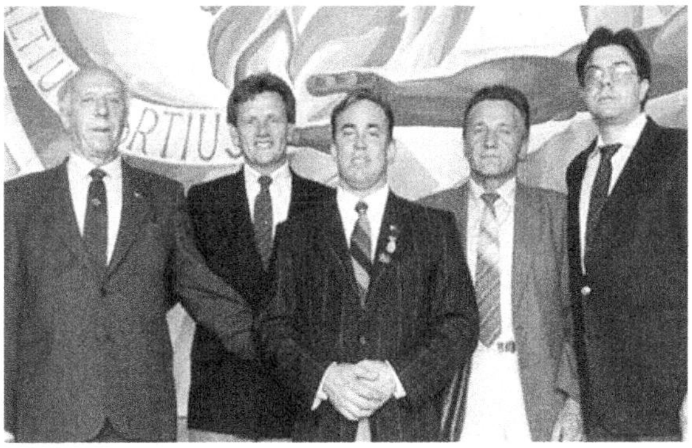

Fig 10 – L-R: Prof Dr. Popov, Drs. Patterson, Stoxen, a Russian MD, the Author at the Institute of Physical Culture in Moscow, 1988

Meeting Dr. Popov

During the arrangements, we had to meet with Prof. Dr. Sergie Popov, at that time Vice-Rector at the Institute. It turned out he was traveling in the US on some mission with the Women's Volleyball team who had recently won the Olympic Gold Medal, and we could meet him at the airport in Pittsburgh, and fly together to Ohio just to talk. We did, and thus began my closest friendship with anyone in Russia.

Despite my getting along so well immediately with Dr. Popov, the arrangements were not to be without setbacks. As it turns out, there was a schism between the factions in Manipulative medicine in the USSR, and they weren't talking to one another. Moreover, they had a movement known as "*Costopravs*", literally Bonesetters, who were traditional or "*barefoot*" doctors, mostly without formal training, though some it seems had really high skill levels. The Manual Therapists, who thought they knew about Chiropractic, and mistakenly equated us with the Costopravs, decided they didn't want Chiropractors at the Institute of Physical Culture, because it might give the Costopravs some credibility and set their cause for recognition back. So they got someone to send a telex to Dr. Enos literally saying that "*we don't want Chiropractors in the Soviet Union. Tell them not to come*". I promptly called my friend Popov and all was resolved, I thought.

In April or May of 1988 we came to Montreal for the 1st time to commence a 24 hour air marathon through Brussels, to Prague, to Bratislava, and finally arriving totally exhausted in then mysterious Moscow, Capital of the "*evil empire*", the Soviet Union.

At that time I knew about five words of Russian, and could not read or write the language. It was really quite scary to be there, completely at the mercy of agents of a government that had a long history of being hostile to my own.

We were received at Sheremetyevo Airport by representatives of the State Sports Committee , known as GOSCOMSPORT. This was the third most powerful Ministry in the USSR after the KGB and the Interior Ministries. Sport was king!

Leaving Sheremetyevo

A bus took us to the Hotel "*Sport*" in the Southwestern part of town, not far from where I would one day buy an apartment. The Hotel was kind of run-down but they did their best to make us feel comfortable there. Each floor had a kind of receptionist/guard, we considered a kind of Cerberus, they called a "*Dezhurnaya*", who had to give you and retrieve your key each time you entered or left. Her job, was also as a kind of morality police, to see that unmarried people of opposite sex didn't go into one another's rooms for monkey business.

It turns out that at that time, there were laws, presumably designed to stem the tide of Prostitution, which made it illegal for a person who resided in say, Moscow, to stay at a Moscow hotel. Nor could unmarried people share a room. You actually had to show your passport (internal or external) to get a room. And at that time, all foreigners had to plan through the notorious KGB associated agency, known as "*Intourist*" to get any accommodations whatever. This allowed the KGB to place an interesting foreigner in a special hotel, presumably one with surveillance facilities, like hidden rooms with two-way mirrors to set up film equipment in the bedrooms, and microphones to eavesdrop on conversations.

Paranoia causes a crash

There were funny stories, like the guy who came on a business trip, and was told about the accommodations. So he brought along de-bugging equipment and in his paranoia, had a tool kit with him. When he arrived in his room, he began searching for suspicious stuff. Coming upon a metal box under his bed he examined it and found that there was a large nut holding it in place.

So he set about loosening the nut. Finally the bolt it held slipped through a hole, and he heard a loud crash below….. it seems he detached the chandelier hanging in the dining room below him!

The Zipperless saga

Our own group was not without its real stories. In each room was a woolen blanket in a quilt cover which instead of having a zipper at one end, had a large hole (about a half meter in diameter), in the center of the top side of the blanket. It took some people a while to realize that this wasn't for them to climb into the cover with their blanket, but merely a replacement for the lack of zippers!

The Lecture

When we all met in the Dining Room that evening, we were introduced to Col. Simeon Raginsky, whom we assumed was a retired KGB officer. His first order of business was to warn us that as we had been required to register all our hard currency when we entered the Country, that we were going to be expected to account for all expenditures while in the Country, and therefore it was "*very illegal to exchange currency in the street*". The reason for this admonition was to become clear in just a few minutes, as we were soon surrounded by teenagers offering to "*exchange currency*", or buy Dollars for Rubles.

To understand the draw to doing this illegally, one has to realize that at that time the Ruble was not an internationally exchanged currency, and the official exchange rate in the banks, known as the "*Golden Ruble*", was $1.50 for each Ruble, or ten Rubles for $15.00.

In the street, these kids were selling Rubles at the rate of 15-20 for each Dollar. That's 20-30 TIMES difference! (by 1991 it would climb to 100/$).

The official rate gave you Soviet money at a rate approximately equal to their own standard of living, and put you on a even par with their economy. Exchanging money on the "*black market*" made you a very wealthy person in comparison to their population.

Naturally, despite Col Raginsky's lecture, most did in fact exchange money with these changers. There was to be another scare at the end of the trip though....

The Spy Gets a Lesson

Every morning, when we met for breakfast, both Col. Raginsky and Prof. Popov would meet me at our own table. I had been assigned my own interpreter too, one Masha Shubnikova, who sat with us.

I was at that time, though still married to Stephanie, already lonely and though I didn't cheat on her, I did occasionally indulge in flirting. And, Masha was kind of cute. It turned out that Col Raginsky spoke fluent French, and Prof Popov, having been stationed in Havana for some eight years, spoke Spanish, so I could converse very well with the Colonel and more or less with Professor Popov, without the benefit of Masha's help.

But, I quickly noticed that whenever I spoke to Raginsky she paid rapt attention, but was obviously bored to death when I spoke Spanish to Popov. I assumed that she spoke French. And later I would ask her about it.

One day we were riding on a bus together and I said, "*Masha, I understand that all the interpreters are trained in a third languages here. What was your third language?"*. She told me that she wasn't really an interpreter at all, but an Attorney, who had worked for the Academy of Sciences, and lost her job because of Gorbachev's "*perestroika*" (restructuring). She had, she said taught herself English. Since she spoke with almost no trace of an accent, I didn't believe her, assuming that she was perhaps militarily trained as a spy, as all the other interpreters had significantly thicker accents than Masha's.

So, for now, I let it go. Still I watched her. It was fun to do so!

Finally, on a trip on the boat touring the Moscow river near the end of our stay, I confronted her again. I entreatied "*Masha, tell me truthfully, you speak French don't you*?" She countered, "*no, why do you think so*?". I said "*first, turn off the microphone*"... she told me to speak openly, that there were no mikes.... So I continued... "*well, Masha, when you next take the KGB spy exam, and you don't want someone to know that you have a language skill... Then, when the subject is speaking, and you pay rapt attention to that language(French), but none when he's speaking the other,(Spanish), it's a dead giveaway*".

A Dressing Down

Then she made a fatal mistake. She said, "*I really don't understand French, I just really like the sound of it*".... So "*say something to me in French*".... Big mistake!

Since she didn't understand it, I could now say ANYTHING to her, no matter how passionate, no matter how intimate! I began to tell her in my best French peppered with all the course argot I knew, how I planned to undress her, and at each portion of her anatomy what I planned to do with her....

In the most graphic, intimate detail! As my dialogue got anatomically lower, and lower, I could see her face getting redder and redder, she was getting really embarrassed! Soon, with smoke coming from her ears, she blurted out "*arrêt-toi*" stop it! (in French). The spy was in from the heat!

We are still friends to this day.... She never forgot me, and we remained in contact.

Great Professors, Great Program

At the renowned Institute of Physical Culture in the Izmailova region of Moscow, we were given our room assignments, twenty DC's and twenty Massage Therapists were there. The faculty we were given was the best in the USSR, one Professor Ilya Verkhoshansky was the man who elucidated plyometric exercise, and another was the famed Vladimir Zatsiorsky, a member of the IOC Medical Commission's, biomechanics Subcommittee. Yet another was the Chief Neurologist of the City of Moscow, Fedin, Anatoly Ivanovich who would the next year become my partner in a *"Joint Venture"* Clinic.

We were thoroughly impressed with the program, our treatment, and the cordiality of the Russian people.

Unparalleled Parallel Processing

The skills of the staff were equally impressive. One interpreter, Elena Pisarchik, was so incredibly skilled that at one lecture we forgot about the poor bastard who was teaching, and started applauding her! It seems she reached a word during a lecture in which she was doing near simultaneous interpreting, which she didn't know. This was odd enough, as she seemed to know what the professors were going to say to us before they said it. But, we then noticed that she had taken out a dictionary and began to make notes. I.e., using her eyes and her hands to do one thing without ever stopping her interpreting, i.e. while her ears and mouth were doing something completely different! An incredible example of parallel processing..... when she began making notes the whole audience composed of some 500 Doctors got up and started applauding HER!.

The Scare at the Airport

When our journey was ending, we all came to the Airport to exit the USSR. Col Raginsky came along for the ride. When all were assembled, he called me aside and asked me in French to explain to the group that "*as he had warned, it was a very serious crime to change money illegally*", and that "*we were going to have to account for all the merchandise we were trying to export from the Soviet Union....*" People were turning all shades of white, realizing that they had no receipts for Rubles, only the merchandise, which clearly was more valuable that the amounts of Rubles for which they could legally account... "*what do we do?*" They all cried... Raginsky went on.... "*so, when you are asked where did you get all these things?.... you reply... it was gifts*"... phewww. So he really was there to run interference for us.

Chapter 9

The Gods of Manipulation

**

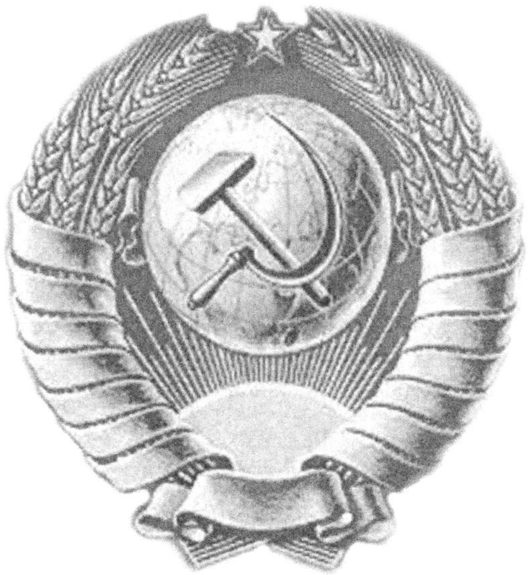

As background, one must understand that as previously alluded to, there were two factions of manual medicine in the USSR. They had a central institute, in Novokuznetsk, in the Urals where they were teaching the techniques, under direction of one Prof. Om Gregorievich Kogan, and a Prof. Ludmila Vasilyeva, both brilliant clinicians and pedagogues, which were akin to Osteopathic methods, i.e. low velocity, high intensity manipulation. This requires much less psychomotor skills than the more in-depth high velocity, low intensity manipulation that constitutes Chiropractic technique.

Until the moment that we arranged to have this symposium, they had never been called to Moscow for such "*recognition*". You see, under the Soviet system this was a bige event for a fledgling profession. So, as we were actually all there, there was some real feelings gratitude towards us for doing this.

Sitel

In our first class, we were introduced to one Dr. Anatoly Boleslavovich Sitel, a pioneer in their manual medicine movement, and chairman of one of the factions which didn't talk to the other. He was, in retrospect the one who didn't want us there in the first place,. Why? Because he obviously had strange idea about what constituted Chiropractic services.

Sitel started by saying, with his nose somewhat in the air..... "*here in the Soviet Union, we are physicians, and before manipulating a patient, we perform a physical examination, perhaps order and read x-ray, and possibly take laboratory tests. Only then do we decide if the patient is a candidate for Manual medicine*". Realizing that this was the cause of the dispute that almost cost us the trip, I jumped in... answering... "*Thank you Professor Sitel. I was so relieved to find that here you too are physicians who examine, diagnose and use lab and x-ray findings to decide the appropriateness of care as we Doctors of Chiropractic do in the United States and elsewhere. I was concerned, because I had heard that (face saving device) here in the USSR there werearefoot doctors who just manipulate everyone who comes to them.*" Whereupon visibly relieved, he gave me a typical Russian bear hug, and shook my hand. Oh how I wish that I had been able to speak directly to him in Russian then!

Sitting in the auditorium at the Institute of Physical Culture, we were presented with some choices for a program, some of which had been left to develop on the fly. So, Dr. Patterson and I considered our possibilities and came up with the idea of a sort of cultural exchange, a round-table discussion and comparison of the techniques they were using, in "*Manualnaya Meditsina*" and Chiropractic.

Manipulation Competition

In the first go around, we were asked to demonstrate our methods of manipulation. So Dr. Popov was recruited as the first "*Victim*" and I proceeded to examine, palpate his neck and finally adjust him. This is a video that one had to see to believe… the tension and the anticipation of that moment… the first official Chiropractic adjustment ever given in the Soviet Union ! He immediately proclaimed that he felt dramatically better and a hush fell over the crowd as they took in what had happened.

Then it fell to one of the Manual manipulators to demonstrate their methods. The patient grimaced for several minutes while he held tension against resistance and obviously caused the patient significant discomfort. In the end the patient also felt somewhat better, but there was a difference that could nearly be measured. Still they didn't concede.

The Phyzli

Then a lady Doctor from Kharkov in Ukraine, came forward and suggested that they had invented an instrument, called a "*Phyzli*", which could measure the electromagnetic energy that was in the body's encompassing field, and that they were using that to test the effectiveness of manipulations.

We accepted the challenge, and they called a young gymnast into the room with a known condition, an acute torticollis or "*wry neck*". Another came in as well and had the same problem. So, we had it, there was one for me and one for them!

We agreed to measure each patient's Phyzli scores before and after each treatment. It was explained that they considered a 10-20% increase in the score a significant success. And the meters had a range of 0-1000 points. They had never seen more than about a 70 point change after their best people manipulated someone.

Each clinician took his turn manipulating. We then measured again. Their patient, treated by the doctor teaching manipulation at one of their post-graduate centers, had a 65 point increase and garnered a standing ovation! Then we measured my patient, who was chattering that her pain was completely gone! There was a 200 point increase.... The room fell totally silent..... then one professor began crying and ran to me putting her arms around my neck and kissing and hugging me.... Crying (through the interpreter)... she said "*Oh my God, you [Chiropractors] are the Gods of manipulation*!"

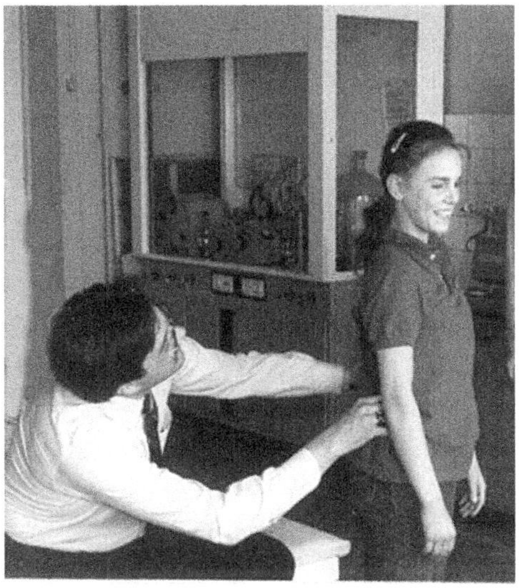

Fig 11 The Author treating Ekaterina Gordeeva

Katya

One afternoon, while at the Institute of Physical Culture, Dr. Popov came over to me and asked "*I hear you have a skating background. Perhaps you would consider consulting in a case of a young skater we have who is suffering from sciatic neuritis*". I was honored to be asked and readily agreed. We went together to another part of the building, and entered a smallish room where there were two women waiting. One a skating official from Canada, and the other an exquisitely beautiful, even angelic young lady of 17 years, sitting facing the doorway. I was sure I knew her, and asked "*don't I know you*?". She replied in English, "*perhaps*"... I said, "*you're Katya, aren't you*?" She just smiled and lit up the room and said "*da*".

Naturally this was Ekaterina Gordeeva, who, together with the man she would later marry, Sergei Grinkov, had just that year before won the Olympic Gold medal in pairs figure skating in Calgary.

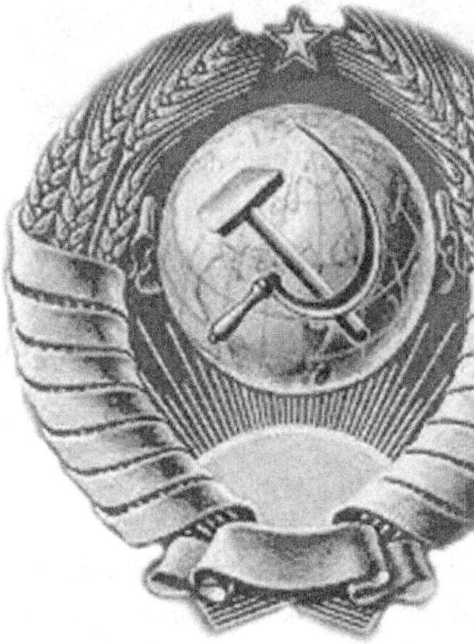

They showed me her films and I performed a physical, orthopedic and neuro exam, and motion palpation, and determined that she had a subluxation in the 5th lumbar level. I asked what had been done to help her and got an entire list of useless therapies. It turned out that she was traveling to New York the next day, and I was leaving two days later, so after I treated her in Moscow, we arranged to meet again in New York. I was given only the name of her coach, and not much else.

When I got home, I ran into New York with no idea how I would find Katya there. But I brought photos of myself with Dr. Popov at the Institute of Physical Culture and with other luminaries I had met there. I figured that this way, if I needed to come to some Soviet agency in the city, they would at least realize that I wasn't just some crank.

I figured right. I found the Soviet mission to the UN, and knocked on their door. It was a dark, forbidding place, with cameras everywhere, and a small cramped waiting room. A receptionist said only "*da*?" And I tried to explain who I was and why I wanted their help. They looked at me like I had three heads coming there like that. But finally someone called an interpreter, and she figured out that I was trying find Katya, and that I was a "*tovarishch*"... comrade! A coach came about an hour later, and we went together to her hotel where she was rooming with Tracy Wilson, the lady who made such a stir in Nagano about the judging corruption while color commentating.

I saw Sergei for the first time, and it was clear to me even then that he was very protective of her, like boyfriend rather than partner. And finally Katya appeared and we got together for treatment on a portable table in her hotel room.

When I returned to Moscow the following year, I was called to the office of the Minister of Sport and given a gold GOSCOMSPORT medal for curing her sciatica and "*saving her career"*. When she wrote her book, I thought it strange that she would forget me and actually mention another Chiropractor she saw here much later.

Chapter 10

A Lawsuit & a Joint-Venture

**

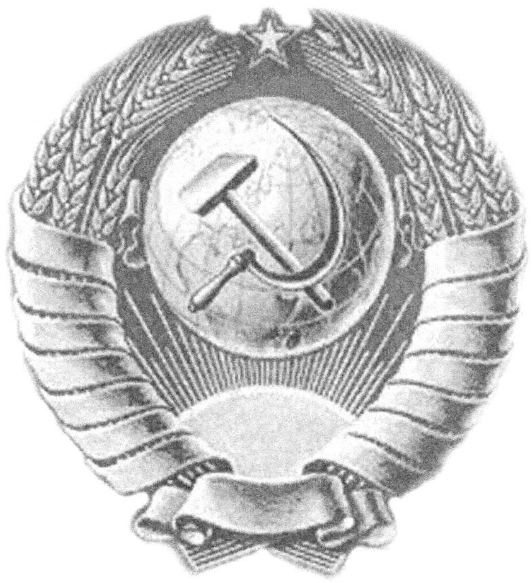

The following year we were invited to send another delegation, a prospect I readily accepted, considering the red carpet treatment we received the first time.

We had laid our plans to get close to the Soviet Sports Committee, as I figured that there was already an official Chiropractor with the US team, the Supreme Council of Olympic Committees of Africa had accepted and recognized FICS, and I assumed that if I could figure out how to get the USSR to officially recognize FICS then the International Olympic Committee (IOC) would be hard pressed to ignore us.

This year we would get to the Headquarters of the State Sports Committee. I just didn't know it would be a Chiropractor having nothing to do with FICS who would walk in there and be mistakenly accepted as one of us.

We were back in the good old USSR, and this time staying not at the Hotel Sport, but at the ABVGD'sky complex (in Russian the first 5 letters of the Cyrillic alphabet are ABVGD) in Ismailova, next to the Institute of Physical Culture. This is where I met Tanya, my 4th wife.

One afternoon at the class arranged at City Hospital no 15, in the region of Vuikhina, on Vyeshnkovkaya Ulitsa, the Professor, Dr. Anatoly Fedin, followed me out to the bus.

With our translator between us, and sitting way in the back for privacy, he suggested in low tones that we form a "*joint-venture clinic*" at his hospital. This was the first in the series of corporate entities that were starting to open up for foreigners to invest in the Soviet economy. Only a few had been opened, and even fewer were profitable. Even so, the temptation of getting a medical license in the USSR and have a full-fledged clinic in a real hospital was really an ego booster.

Investors

I agreed to try to raise the capital and on my return home, found willing souls interested in the same ideas, and each with $25,000 to invest in it. What they would get, was bragging rights to ownership in a clinic at a hospital in Moscow, a license to practice medicine in the Soviet Union, a tee-shirt with a logo, and possibly, just possibly some profits, if this thing actually made money.

Coming back in just six weeks, after raising about $250,000 Dollars, for the first time I found myself without an officially provided interpreter. I had only Tanya. I quickly realized that I would need to be able to communicate in Russian by myself or Tanya would be my only lifeline. I realized that I couldn't read "*Men*" or "*Women*". This could be dangerous, and embarrassing! At this stage, I still tried to trust that the girl who said "*I love you*" wouldn't hurt my prospects here. That trust would be short-lived, but at that point it was still strong.

Remember that Tanya WAS an interpreter, even simultaneously qualified, and thus a very good partner to have on my side in this matter. She went everywhere with me. But there were even then problems. She would periodically insist on saving me money by forcing me to spend hours food shopping at somewhere like Yelisevsky's in Rubles instead of spending dollars and getting my food shopping done in minutes at the Irish House Supermarket. Or walking for many blocks to use the metro, rather than flag down a taxi who would demand a few dollars from an obvious foreigner but save hours in walking time.

Cheat Anyone You Can

The system was really fraught with traps for the unwary. And there was no way to be prepared for everything. Nearly everyone was dishonest... the system seemed to be "*take what you can right now. Forget that you might want to do business with these people later, because later might never come. The regime might come back anytime.*" Even the government was in on this. And their rules were so incredibly complex, and primitive that there frequently seemed to be no rhyme or reason for any of them except to make people's lives that much harder.

Food Shopping Nightmare

Food shopping was an exercise in Kafkaesque deliberate disorganization. At the classiest Russian food market, Yelisevsky's, one stood in one line for kolbasa (salami), another for eggs, and so on.... This wasn't bad enough.... When you got to the counter, and told them how much of the product you wanted, the salesperson gave you a little slip of paper, with a number on it and tells you to go to the cashier's line to pay for it. Then after that line, you got a receipt, and could come back to the food product line AGAIN, to finally retrieve your whatever. It could easily take all day to go food shopping for a few basic staples.

The National Pastime

My partner was no exception. It was clear to me from the gitgo that he was no one to be trusted, and he quickly proved me right. He was in this to steal everything he could get his hot little hands on, and the hell with the investors. But, I had to continue the game, because I had committed myself with my colleagues who gave me their money.

Right away we had to pay out more for everything then we had planned in the beginning. There were hidden charges everywhere. If we planned a seminar, and had to pay the university for example, then we had an estimate from them for x amount, but when we got a bill, it was for y. What were the differences? Well, we had agreed to pay for a room, and faculty, but we hadn't figured for rental of the desks, erasers, and chalk! What about the heat and electricity? Then oh yes, we forgot about the lady who had to come in and clean the next day… and probably she needs lunch?

It was really like this… every negotiation was that way. It frankly got really infuriating at times, and on a couple of meetings I nearly walked out and told him where to go… that turned out to be a good tactic, because when he saw I was totally infuriated, he'd back off and tell me that it was ok, he'd deal with it.

Notaries were royalty

Finally we got to actually registering a corporation. There were two lawyers, an accountant, and then we had to go to a Notary. In the US, practically anyone can be a notary, unless you're a convicted felon. Not so elsewhere. In the Soviet Union, you had to be first trained as a lawyer or accountant, then VOLUNTEER your time for some six months at an existing Notary office, and finally take an exam. If you passed, you were placed on a list, which of course presumably you could bribe your way on to the top of. Then when called you could be a notary.

At the end of the USSR period, the notaries were making a relative fortune in bribes to handle the requests for signing corporate papers, bank cards, and the like. The alternative to paying bribes was to stay on lines for weeks at a time. Literally.

We met one day to finalize the corporate entity we were known as a *"sovmesto predpriatie, actsioneernovo obshchestvo, zakritovo typa"* … I had to learn this…. It means *"Joint venture, stock issuing company, closed type"* There were other variants. But we had specific investors who held the only shares. So we were this form.

Tailoring a copy

I was given a Xerox copy of the Corporate charter, in which I was named President of the US filial (affiliate), and VP of the Soviet filial, and Fedin the opposite. I assumed initially that having a copy of my corporate documents was all the proof I needed, as in this Country that I was an officer. Ha! In that system, copies of documents were absolutely invalid, unless they were with original signatures and signed and sealed by a notary. The notary actually had to sew the document together with a needle and thread, and then place his/her seal over the knots. Then the copy gave you authority.

The Round Seal

Then there was the little matter of a seal. It seems that every obshchestvo, i.e., legal entity had to have a round seal, to be used only with purple ink. No seal, no authority, even with a sewn copy of the charter. He with the seal wins. Naturally, there were enormous impediments to getting such a seal made at that time. It was criminal to reproduce them without permission, read "*license*" from the Militia (Police). That took reports that the seal was stolen or lost and etc., etc., weeks of lines and kneeling at the feet of those in power. Fedin told us in front of my lawyer that one could only have one seal. It was another lie. I already had found out that an obshchestvo could have two of them. And, best of all, I had a driver with a connection who for forty dollars could duplicate it for me. I actually had it in my briefcase when we went to Fedin to discuss getting another seal.

You should have been there! He went into this whole song and dance about "*getting a license for the seal, applying to the militia etc, etc... it should take weeks, and unfortunately you have to leave on Monday... if only you could stay a couple of weeks longer... boo hoo*". I replied that, "*here's a copy of the new law which says we can have another seal made at our request"....* "*So, we are agreed that I can have one made*?"... Convinced that it would take me weeks to get one, he agreed. I then said, "*so, that being done, do you want to use your seal, or mine to officialize this agreement*?" And took my seal out.... I thought he'd fall off his chair.

Bank Cards

Then there was the matter of a bank card. You know, the signature card one easily signs at any bank? In the USSR, one had to get an appointment with a bank officer by phone to arrange to be met at the bank door to obtain blank cards. Then one had to get all the parties whose signatures would be "*legalized*" by the notary, to come together to the notary office and then pay something like 100.00 US$ for each signature on each card. This was the going bribe amount then in vogue.

So, I asked Fedin why my name wasn't on the bank card? He told me that it could be but there was a limit to the number of people who could have access to a bank account. Wrong! Lie! Bell... Whistle! I already new all about the bank cards, because on that trip into Moscow, I was in Business Class, and as luck would have it, I was sitting next to the Minister of Finance of Russia, and we talked for some five or six hours about world affairs, etc. He told me that he was also the President of the Bank in which we happened to have opened the account, and "*if I had any trouble to call him anytime*". So, when Fedin told us in the first get together that trip that it was impossible to get my name on the bank card, I already knew it was not. As I left his office, I called my new friend at the bank, and was told to come over. Whereupon he handed me a batch of blank bank cards to fill in as required (at a notary of course).

Next meeting with Fedin , were told that he'll "*get a bankcard for me, and the next time I'm in Moscow we can get them signed*". I suggested that I "*would go and get the cards myself, now*". He answered that that "*would be impossible as I needed to have propusk (pass) just to get in the front door. You won't even be admitted onto the territory of the bank he said.*". He even seemed very sincere this time. So, I said, "*well, in any case, if I can get the cards, he'd arrange to go with me to the notary?*". Sure of his position this time, and never dreaming that I could have had such a powerful friend, he agreed readily. I then said, "*ok.... So here's the needed card ! Let's go!*" I really thought he'd lose it.... This time he got a new respect for my connections and was starting to have a little fear for playing with me. He knew of course, the level of power that it took to get those cards, and it made him think twice next time.... But not three times... he still tried to steal and eventually succeeded in taking control of the company, but not before I made another connection, which would prove more profitable for me in the long run.

Penny Wise and Pound Foolish

He actually would have made a lot more money with this clinic, had he been honest with us, then this way. He got a few dollars but lost in the long run.. Penny wise and pound foolish. It seemed the norm there, then.

After several attempts to resolve the irregularities, it became apparent that there was no way to make this thing profitable for anyone but Fedin. And we abandoned our hopes of making money at the Hospital.

During the process however, we had a couple of really good times there. Once such came when some of the American investors came to town to see the facilities. We took them on a tour of Moscow, and some of the surrounding towns and villages, Like Suzdal, Zagorsk, and Vladimir; what are known as part of the "*Golden Ring*". On the way to Suzdal, we were supposed to stop at some restaurant on the highway to eat.... But we were in the middle of a blizzard, and it was closed. Soon we saw a roadside stand barbecuing chicken (or I like to think it was chicken).... In any event, it was the most delicious poultry I ever tasted..... In Suzdal, they make a beer with honey, called something very close to mead. Myawd it's pronounced. Also incredible.

Slavyansky Bazaar

One night, Fedin decides to take us all to the famous dinner theatre, Slavyansky Bazaar. Being the official Chief Neurologist for the City, he had some power there too. We got served a banquet fit for a Tsar. Caviar at each place, both Red and Black. Champagne, Cognac, and Wine at every place... real crystal.. and the course just kept coming out... it seemed never to end. I assumed that he'd pick up the tab. After all he had a relatively large amount of our money already. Several thousand dollars. But still he hands me the bill and tells me... "*these are the foreign investors, so you have to pay for this*." Remember the exchange rates? Remember that we were now getting about 100 Rubles for the dollar in the street, and it was still 1.5 Rubles to the Dollar in the Bank. Initially scared at being stuck with his bill, it was really hard to keep from laughing at the prices... official rates charged because of Fedin's contacts. About 1300 Rubles... a lot of money if I had exchanged in the banks... but for me, just $13.00 total... $1.00/person !!!

An Interloper

All the time we were in Moscow, on our second excursion, working to get in the front door at GOSCOMSPORT, we were unaware of it, but another DC was by coincidence in Moscow. We were working at cross purposes and neither knew about the other.

FICS was still in its infancy, and lots of DC's had never heard about us. One such guy was a Doctor from the Minneapolis-St Paul area. Dr. Zhuk, we'll call him, was originally from Kiev, in Ukraine. A Jewish immigrant, he had finished school at the Kiev Institute of Physical Culture, which gave him the equivalent of something between a masters and a bachelors degree in physical education by our standards. Once here, he went to Chiropractic school and became a DC.

By the time of this occurrence, the Chiropractic profession had developed a post-graduate, board certification program in Sports Medicine, called *"Certified Chiropractic Sports Physician."* Dr. Zhuk was not Board Certified or even Board eligible at that time. In fact he was not even advertising that he treated sports injuries.

Also, at this period in history, an organization opened by President Eisenhower, called the *"People to People Ambassador Program"*, was in full swing. In this program, the idea was to bring together people of various professions, with their counterparts in certain Countries, like China and the USSR. It worked like a glorified travel agency, sending thousands of invitations to people in each profession, saying things like *"YOU have been chosen to represent your Country in the People to People, as an Ambassador for Chiropractic."* Maybe a few hundred were sent out, the idea being to see if anyone wants to pay the few thousand to go and be able to say they're an *"Ambassador."* Naturally there is no official ambassadorial title to this, but people like to think they are something special and many fall for the approach. Dr. Zhuk wanted to go, he had a second reason. His mom and dad divorced when his mother took him to the US and he hadn't seen his dad for years. They were going to be in Kiev, and ended up in Moscow.

Understand, no one in Chiropractic had selected this guy to represent the profession. No Chiropractic organization had any voice in this. He basically selected himself, when he accepted the sales pitch from the P to P program.

So this self selected *"Ambassador"* (without portfolio) is traveling around the USSR, representing to the Soviet medical profession that he's some kind of *"official ambassador*" for the Chiropractic profession and no one here knows that he's doing this!

He turns up in Moscow at the same time we do. Only "*we*" are an official delegation selected by the World's Chiropractic associations to represent them to the Soviet Sports Committee. Then, while we are in Ismailova, at the National Institute of Physical Culture, and the Minister is getting ready to invite us to Committee headquarters; in walks Dr. Zhuk, blissfully unaware of our presence, work, or mission as the official delegation for the profession, nor our two years and tens of thousands of dollars investment in this project, and presents himself at the headquarters of the Sports Committee at exactly the moment that they wanted our delegate to come over!! They naturally assumed he was with us. Never imagining that it could be such a coincidence, he's invited up to the office of the Deputy Minister of Sport, and since he speaks Russian, and they told us he represented to them that he was an "*Internationally known sports Chiropractor*", a title, considering his lack of Boards in Sports Chiropractic, and his failure to even advertise himself as treating sports injuries, he appears to have just made up at the spur of the moment. And, they love it! Dr. Zhuk thus gets invited, much to his surprise and delight, to serve as the team doctor, for the Goodwill Games to be held that season in Seattle, WA.

FICS doesn't hear about it until it hits the Chiropractic papers. Naturally this miracle for him is a career changer! He's bragging from the rooftops about his good fortune. And we are left in the dark as to why we never got to see the Minister of Sport?

When the story breaks, as I was the FICS representative in Moscow, the board calls me and asks me "*who is this guy*?" and, "*why don't you know where he came from*?".

Also, by the time the story broke here, I had been appointed Chief Physician to the Olympic Team and due to our inquiry they un-appointed him to further events. In fact they really shut the door on him, despite my efforts to ask that they do it politely and diplomatically.

What I only much later found out, was that when I was appointed, the Minister forgot, or just didn't bother, to tell their own Chief Physician that he had been replaced. So, this was the one guy who hated me there, and for reasons understandable from his perspective.

So, when Dr. Zhuk shows up in Moscow for the next event they invited him to, they didn't even meet him at the airport. In fact, I later heard that no one but the Russian Doc who got booted, would talk to him. But, that guy tells him, not that Press was a delegate of an International agency representing Zhuk's own profession, but that "*Press probably had you booted out of professional jealousy*" ! Of course Zhuk is furious!

He returns to the US in an abysmal funk and runs to a lawyer to file a Slander/Libel action against me personally, and against his own profession's International Agency, FICS. And naturally the very member of the FICS' Board who told me to intercede, and who vetted my letter, was the one who later used it against me, trying to hurt my relationship with the other members of the Board of the very agency I founded. Saying "*look what Press got us into?*" Imagine the irony?

During the discovery phase of the lawsuit, my insurance carrier's lawyer figures that we may actually have to go to Moscow to try the case under Russian law. Because everything happened there! So, despite that the Russian doctor who told Zhuk about me, dies in his soup during the process, and despite that Zhuk never knows it; the insurance company decides it's cheaper to give him a few thousand dollars to go away than go to Russia to try the case. Even though his only witness was dead, and the whole case was based only on a wounded ego, and that we were virtually assured to prevail.

Chapter 11

"Dr. Press, It's a problem"

**

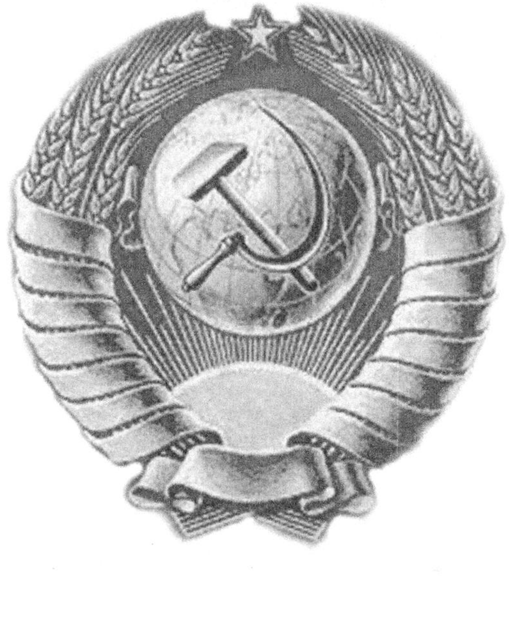

On leaving Moscow, the delegation continued as the previous year, on to the beautiful Venice of the North, St. Petersburg, before attempting to leave by way of Talinn, in Estonia, and thence by ferry across the Baltic to Helsinki, Finland.

The prior year, we had been billeted at the lovely Leningrad Hotel, on the Neva River in the heart of town. As we were leaving the train station, where we were greeted by a beautiful young pediatrician, moonlighting as an interpreter, Anna Boldisheva, we started towards town. As Chef-de-Mission, I was the one whose job it was to resolve problems, so when I realized we weren't heading in the right direction for the Leningrad, I inquired with Anna. "*oh*" she exclaimed, "*Dr. Press, there's a problem*". This was to become the recurrent theme throughout our stay in "*Peterburg*".

"*What's the problem?*", I asked .... "*well*" she said, "*We're not staying at the Leningrad*". "*Oh?*", I allowed.... "*well, there was a fire there, and they aren't putting up foreigners now*". "*OK*", I said, "*then where re we staying?*". "*I can't tell you*" she murmured...."*huh?*".... I choked a bit.... "*What do you mean*?" I went on.... "*we have to know where we're staying, because, these are important internationally known people, and they have to notify their offices where they can be reached*".

Hotel without a name

She became pensive, and then, after some reflection, "*well, we're staying at the hotel without a name*". I said, "*Anna, that's not good enough dear. We need to be able to tell our people where we're staying!*" ... "*Oh ok, I guess it's ok to tell you.... It's a dormitory attached to the Institute for Nuclear Physics Research, but you have to understand that under the laws of the Soviet Union, Nuclear Physics, officially doesn't exist, thus a hotel without a name!*". I successfully held back a laugh.

At the Hotel-without-a-name, we were shown to our rooms. A lovely quaint, and cozy little place, all brand new then, the rooms were also by comparison to Moscow, really nice. Then we tried to wash. No hot water! I called Anna. "*Dr. Press, we have a problem*"..... "*well..... you see not every hotel has it's own heat and hot water heater system. There's a regional plant that produces heat and hot water for the entire area, and every Spring and Summer they pick a region at a time to shut down for maintenance for two weeks, and this is our two weeks!*". "*So*", I inquired, "*no hot water for the duration*?" "*Right*".

OK.... Ingenuity to the rescue. I knew that there was likely a "*Vernisage*" (flea market) on weekends somewhere nearby. So, I sent an errand boy from the Hotel-without-a-name to the market with funds to buy us five Samovars, and some charcoal briquettes. We set them up in the corridors near the window and heated our own hot water. It was really quite quaint.

We left for Dinner, which was supposed to take place at the Jazz Club. Located in an old Czarist building, the theatre holds around 500 people and it was sold out. We were seated in really nice seats at a table, and waited for dinner and the show. An hour and a half later, and still no food. I went to Anna. She came back in ten minutes, and said...."*Dr. Press, we have a problem*".

The Chef Died

I thought, "*what now*?"... She said, "*there'll be no dinner here tonite*". I had to ask "*why?*". She said.. "*the chef died*". I was laughing, and feeling guilty at the same time.. after all maybe someone had actually died.... She stopped me... "*it's not funny, the chef really did die!*".... she said seriously. I couldn't believe that there was ONE chef for 500 people... but we went to the Leningrad for a late dinner. At least their restaurant was still open.

Next morning, we were scheduled for classes at the famous Lesgaft Institute, the St Petersburg version of the National Institute of Physical Culture. We had scheduled the full day for Monday, because last year, we were in Petersburg and Monday was our only day off, and all the museums and palaces are closed on Mondays! So this year I was wiser and prepared for that. Tuesday morning, we had a half-day of classes, and it had been raining all morning, and I feared that we wouldn't be able to get the rocket boat to Petrodvoretz (Peter's Palace) otherwise known as the Summer Palace.

After class, we headed to the pier. There was no boat and no one in sight. I turned to Anna... and asked her to find out about the boat. After about 15 minutes she came back and I could predict what I would hear.... "*Dr. Press, we have a problem*". I couldn't hold it in now.... I said, "*Did the Captain die*?". She, already realizing the black comedy in this, said "*sort of*!". I said "*what is happening here*?". She explained that because the water was a bit rough due to the rain, there were no other tourists here, and the Captain didn't want to take this big boat the 45 minutes ride to Petrodvoretz with only the six of us! What to do?

Buying the Boat

I asked Anna, "*how many seats are on the boat*?". "*50*", I asked "*how much are the tickets?*" She said... "*5 Rubles each*". Recalling that we were illegally changing money in the streets, and that to her each Ruble was a $1.50, the seats were relatively expensive in her mind at officially $7.50 each! So, when I suggest that we buy all 50 seats, she was thinking the Russian equivalent of 50 X $7.50...$375.00 !! perhaps a year and a half's salary for her. To us however, exchanging in the black market, the Ruble was about $.01 each, and thus the whole boat actually cost us $2.50 to rent completely. So, when I told her "*here's the 250 Rbls., go buy all 50 tickets*", I thought she'd faint.

Now that we had established ourselves as the rich Americans, we got our private boat. The trip was uneventful to the Palace grounds and we even had an interpreter sent with us to tell us about the place on the trip over. When we arrived at the Island pier, another young man approached us to tell that he would be our guide at the actual palace area. We began the rather long walk towards the Palace, when I realized we were leaving the Palace off to the right and heading away from the building complex. I said "*young man, we want to go that way...*" he replied, "*that's towards the Palace*". I said, "*I know, we want to see the Palace first*". He said, "*oh that's impossible... the Palace closes at 1:00PM and its already 12:30... you'll never get into the Palace now... the guards go off duty*". I must have glared at him, because he was visibly upset.... I, on the other hand was really furious... how could this have happened? A second trek to St Petersburg only to be cheated again out of seeing the Palaces? Again due to oversight of the schedules? I was more than furious, I was devastated.... But, ingenuity took over.... I handed him twenty US dollars (I knew this could buy them 2000 Rubles, or $3000.00 US Dollars worth at official rates)... imagine! I said, "*go find the manager of the ticket sales... tell him or her, that you are with a delegation of famous Doctors sent here by the Kremlin and that this is the second time we have come to see the Palace and are being turned away... that our hosts at the Kremlin will be furious when we call Moscow.*".

Buying the Palace

In 15 minutes he comes back. "*I can't believe it! I can't believe it!* " He was yelling... "*for twenty dollars, you have bought the Palace! You have free run of the place and there will be no guards!... I guess you can take what you like. No one will be there to stop you.*"... I assured him that we would do no such thing. We got to spend a leisurely unsupervised time in the Palace and simply locked the door behind us as we left. In retrospect, had we been dishonest people, we could have tried to filch something… but we do have to sleep at night.

As we arrived back at the pier to leave for town, we see a long line of locals waiting to board the ferry. I asked our guide why they were not admitted to the boat? He told me, "*well, you bought all the seats, so you own the boat, and they won't allow anyone else to occupy your seats*". I asked how they would get back to town without this boat? It was the last boat, I was told and the trip back could take several hours, of walking, and then busses and trains. I conferred with my delegation and we decided to invite as many as could fit on the boat to board as our guests…. The applause was deafening…. The Russians, understanding what had transpired, carried me onto the boat on their shoulders shouting , roughly… "*hurrah for the rich Americans*". I was Donald Trump for $7.50 !!

Train to Talinn

Next morning we boarded the train again. This time headed for Talinn, Estonia. We were really looking forward to seeing this beautiful ancient city on the Baltic, but my anticipation was squelched by my trepidation about the fact that the Baltic States were in the throes of a schism with the Soviet Union and we didn't know when that could begin, or if there would be shooting. It turned out to be that morning as we were arriving they chose to split!

On the train, our interpreter Tatiana Schach, was surly as usual. I asked her who was meeting us at the train station, to interpret. She replied that we would have an Estonian girl there working for us. I asked her if she spoke any Estonian herself?.. She replied "*They all must speak Russian*".

Back home, at my Masonic Lodge, one of our members is one K Jaak Roosare, an Estonian National and attorney who had been Vice-President of the Estonian American

Federation, and spoke the language fluently. Hearing that I was headed there, he had given me the heads up that they were preparing to secede soon. And he tried to teach me some Estonian.... No mean trick, this is an extremely difficult language indeed.

But I knew enough to greet the interpreter and ask in Estonian if she spoke Russian or English.... So I told Tanya Schach what Jaak told me. Also, that due to the impending secession, the Estonians were feeling none too friendly towards the Russians this day.

She insisted that "*they all speak Russian*"... So I let it go....

When we arrived in Talinn, a beautiful young lady appeared and was greeted in Russian by Tanya... "*Zdrastvuite*" (hello), she said. The Estonian girl completely ignored her.

She tried again.... "*Zdrastvuite...*" she tried, to no avail. I stepped in and said... "*meene olan Ameriklaner, kas te oskate Vene keelt?*" *("I'm an American, do you speak Russian?")* She turned to me, smiled and said "*for you... Da*". Tanya was furious and ashamed.

Estonian Revolution Begins....

We had left the lovely Anna behind in Petersburg, but thanks to the start of what would turn out to be a bloodless revolution, the trend continued in Talinn.

As we start to town, our Estonian guide tells me that we will have only a few hours in their city. When I inquire why? She relates that they are seceding from the USSR and the Estonians are closing the port, so if we dally, we won't be able to get out of Estonia, and she didn't know when we could leave again. Oh my...

OK... I had business at their now, National Olympic Committee Headquarters, so I headed for that venue while my compatriots went into town. I soon got a call, to get right to the port, it seems they were planning to close up, and not allow even our ferry to leave for Helsinki, thus stranding not only our six doctors, but about a hundred Finns to boot.

I asked when they thought we could leave Estonia? They said it could be several weeks! So, I called my friend at the Olympic Committee Headquarters and he promised to try to help us.... A few minutes later a call came through.... Moscow would be really pissed, they said if we were kept as hostages to the revolution. They decided to let our ferry leave, and again I was carried onto the boat. This time by happy Finns....

Chapter 12

The Cardboard Coup

**

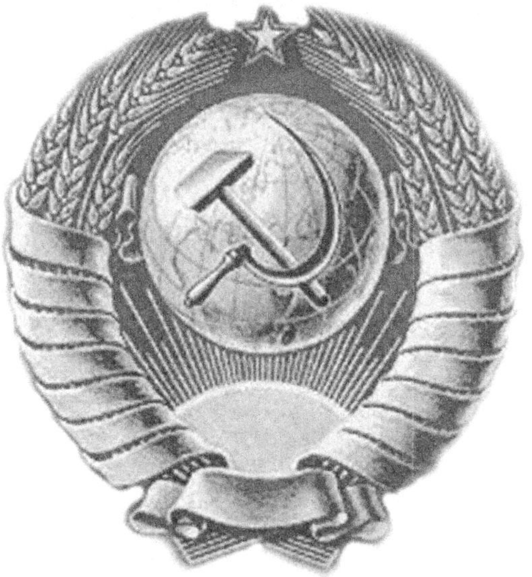

It was the start of the Russian Winter in 1991, and Yeltsin had been elected President of Russia, though Mikhail Gorbachev was Chairman of the Communist party and still in the Kremlin. The Red Soviet flag still flew above the Kremlin gates.

Gorbachev was negotiating a new Soviet constitution. Everyone was upset by this. The leaders of the 15 Republics, (Russia, Georgia, Azerbaijan, etc.) were unhappy because they weren't being given enough autonomy, and the hard core, hard-liners; Boris Pugo, Interior Minister; Kryushkov, Chairman of the KGB and Yanaev, Party Vice-Chairman, got together to plan a coup.

I firmly believe that Gorbachev knew they would do this, and tried to take advantage of their zealotry.

What Mikhail Sergeievich Gorbachev really wanted was to have the Soviet Union do what China is doing today. I.e., maintain a strong "*Socialist*" center, and still allow private business to flourish. It was not to be, thanks to the upstart Yeltsin. But how did Yeltsin get this chance?

Twice before, Chairmen had been spirited away from their seats of power, and each time it was when they went to their Dacha's during critical times like these. Gorbachev certainly knew that those who fail to learn from history are condemned to repeat it. And still at just this critical moment, he goes to his dacha.

Recall Eduard Shevardnadze, who was Gorbachev's closest friend for many years? He was coincidently the first to run from the Party, "*Chicken Little*" like... claiming that a "*Putsch (coup) was coming*"...

I believe that he and Gorbachev arranged to play "*good cop, bad cop*" with the hard liners.... Gorby being the "*good Commy*" and Shavardnadze the turncoat, who was now free to plan with the more liberal generals to avoid a take-over in the event of a real coup attempt, and report back to his pal in the Kremlin.

Tanya was still in Moscow when Yanaev and his "*emergency committee*" had Gorbachev surrounded in his dacha, by the presidential guard.... What a joke! I fail to believe that the entire presidential guard, all Gorbachev's hand-picked guys, was really under the direction of the coup plotters...

Gorbachev however, was taking no chances... he apparently had not one, but two videos pre-taped to use in the event that his plans went awry.... They would, but not in the direction he planned.

Once the putsch began, and the tanks, driven by Russian boys, not Azeris, or Kazakhs, who would not have had much trouble shooting at Russians, drove into Moscow, it was clear that the coup was a bust. But why?

First of all the Chairman of the KGB and the Interior Ministry didn't know that they would have to cut off communications? Cut the CNN feed; close Sheremetyevo Airport; stop radio and tv broadcasts, except for what they wanted to show????

It's a ridiculous assumption. Moreover, that the military sent in Russian boys, presumably to blow up all the demonstrators and sweep away the bodies, and that this could all have been on CNN for the world to watch???

When the tanks came rolling into town, and I saw the Babushkas yelling at the Russian boys driving with the tank hatches UP, not to do this, that there had been "*enough Russian blood spilled*".... And the Tank drivers calling back "*don't worry, nothing's going to happen*".... Finally, it was CNN who reported that when Boris Pugo, Yanaev and

Kryushkov met at Lyubyanka Prison (KGB Headquarters), and presented their plans to the mid-level management, majors, captains, colonels, etc.... how to kill all the protesters, clean up the mess afterwards, etc, etc. The mid-level people just said "*forget it*" and went and sat in the basement of Lyublyanka until the crisis was over. Frankly, I count them as the real heroes of the Putsch.

It was at this critical juncture, when Gorbachev was still out of touch, and Yeltsin was available, that he climbed onto one of the tanks and the youth of Moscow brought all their BMW's and other newly minted symbols of capitalism, and parked around the tanks for the world to see, and they rallied for freedom.... And Yeltsin seized the moment, and the rest is as we say, History. The hard liners had been given enough rope to hang themselves, and they did exactly that.... Either Pugo or Kryushkov killed himself, and the other was imprisoned with Yanaev as traitors. Yeltsin moved into the Kremlin, and the whole Soviet Union collapsed around him.

Later, on one of my numerous trips back and forth, I sat with one of Gorbachev's press secretaries for the 10 plus hours of the flight to New York City, and although he couldn't "*confirm or deny*"... ha, ha.... He just smiled verrry broadly, and said "*maladyetz*" (good for you!).

Chapter 13

The Meeting with Samaranch

**

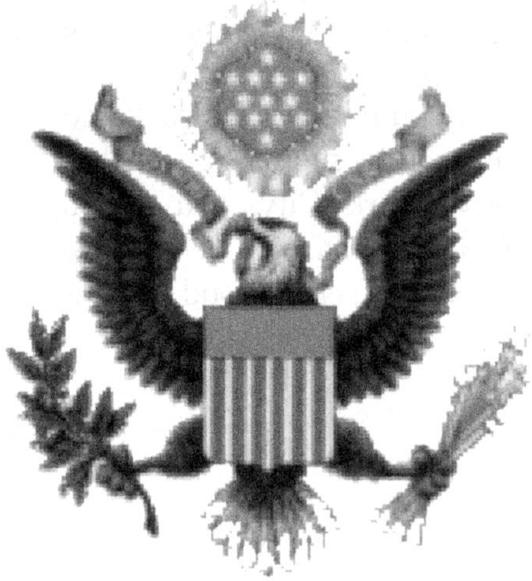

The Summer of 1989, the FICS determined to meet in the eternal city, Rome. It was gorgeous there that time of year, though quite hot. We were in the midst of negotiations with the staff of H.E., Juan Antonio Samaranch, President of the International Olympic Committee, for a face-to-face in at the Présidence of the IOC in Lausanne.

Rome

Through the auspices of a DC in Calgary, who had actually volunteered to work as Mr. Samaranch's chauffeur during the Winter Games there in 1988, we were promised such a meeting. And, we had it timed to occur right after our Congress in Rome. Perfect! We could meet, discuss our approach, and run up to Lausanne for "*the meeting*". At the Congress in Rome, I was still presiding officer. The Board held a private meeting behind the scenes and it was decided, promoted by the already forming clicque of Pierson, Patterson, et al, that it was too important to allow just one person to hold the meeting alone. I was mandated to take at least one member of our Board with me.

Ok, we agreed that either [17]Dr. Daniele Bertamini, of Italy, or [18]Dr. Benet-Canut of Mexico, would come along. I was all for that, because I understood that Samaranch was from Barcelona and his first language was Catalan, and Benet, being Catalunian spoke perfect Catalan.

They were both going off on respective trips. Bertamini to a skiing trip in the Italian alps, and Benet-Canut to some relative in Spain. Both assured me that they would be available on a moment's notice to run up to meet me in Lausanne if called.

---

[17] then President of the Associazione Italiani di Chiropractici, current President of the Fédération Internationale de Chiropratique du Sports

[18] President of the Associacion Mexicana de Quiropractica, A.C., then member of the Executive Board of the Fédération Internationale de Chiropratique du Sports, and the World Federation of Chiropractic.

Dr. Patricia Arthur, of Hawaii, who was one of the Chiropractic plaintiffs in the Wilk et al, v AMA et al, Federal lawsuit that opened up the health professions to the joint practice of DC's and MD's was our treasurer then. She stayed with me waiting for the call from Lausanne. It was about two to three days after the FICS Congress ended when we got from Ani Inchauspé, Samaranch's secretary "*come straight up to Lausanne the next day*". No notice.

I desparately called for Benet-Canut and failed to find him. I tried every number he gave me, but to no avail. I tried calling Bertamini's number too. No answer! I tried his home and office, but they just told me he was incommunicado in the Alps. No luck and time was running out. I was desperate.... I really didn't want to violate my mandate, but I also could not afford for FICS to lose the opportunity to meet with Samaranch.

I called Dr. Christoph Diem, in Switzerland, past president of the Swiss Chiropractic Association, and President of the World Federation of Chiropractic, for advice. He suggested taking a Dr. Robert of Geneva with me instead. I tried the others again and got nowhere. So, Jean Robert came with me to Samaranch's office.

Benet-Canut never forgave me. He tells that he called the hotel and was told despite that I was staying there at the time, that I had "*checked out*". Piffle.

Tête-à-tête

The meeting was momentous for us. Samaranch was really a great gentleman. He gave us nearly 45 minutes of his precious time. Far more than many heads of state have received. His concerns were mainly procedural; i.e, to run it through his Medical Commission, i.e, Prince De Merode, with whom we had already gotten nowhere. This was a

Belgian, and the Belgian's were, with the French the most anti-Chiropractic societies in the World.

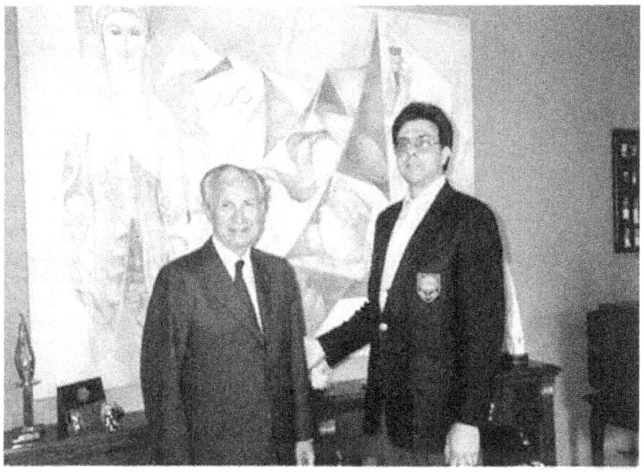

Fig 12 the Author (R) with H.E., Juan Antonio Samaranch at the Présidence of the IOC, in Lausanne

I demurred.. Finally, saying, frankly Your Excellency, "*I have some concerns about doing that.*" Samaranch inquired what my problem was?.... I said.."*Well, Your Excellency, let's hypothesize that tomorrow you were to decide to create an Olympic Clergy commission. Would you decide yourself which religions to include, or would you call the Vatican to determine this for you?*" He just nodded in understanding... still nothing immediate came of it all.... He still gave it to the Medical Commission, and as of the date of his retirement, they had simply never bothered to answer him! Certainly this was behind his decision to allow a pilot project in Australia at the Summer Games in Sydney despite their intransigence.

Chapter 14

The Winter Olympic Games

**

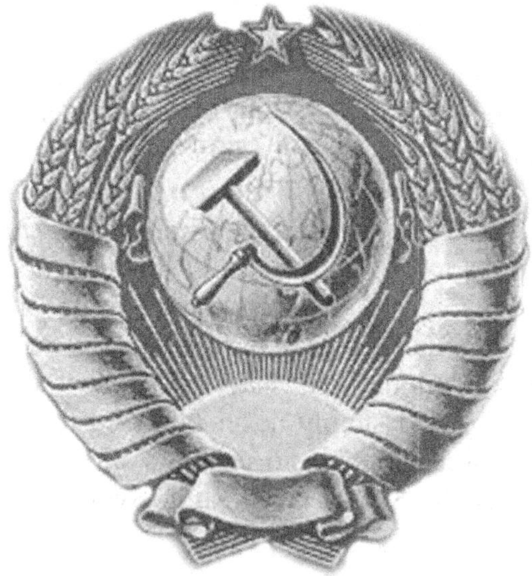

Sometime in the Summer of 1990, while we were in the throes of developing the Clinic, I got another call from the office of the Minister of Sport of the Soviet Union. "*Come to the GOSCOMSPORT headquarters, please*".

When I arrived, they had a few dignitaries present, and the Minister told me, "*since you were able to help our Champion, Katya Gordeeva, and since you have worked with other sportsmen here and been such a help, we would like to recognize your profession's Federation (FICS), and ask them to nominate a Doctor to come with our Olympic team to Albertville next year*". I replied that I would have "*to discuss that with our Board of Directors*", and "*get back to him*".

When I arrived at my flat in Belyaevo, I called Dr. Pierson in California, and there was a conference call with others which ensued. I was called back and told, "*you're our guy in the USSR, you're it!*". So, I gave him the fax number of the Minister's Office, and asked him to fax that directly to the Minister, "*so it wouldn't look like I nominated myself*".

The next day, I again received a call from Minister Rusak's secretary, and was again asked to appear at headquarters.

Chief Physician

When I arrived, there were fewer people around, but the Minister said, "*Thank you for coming Dr. Press. When I spoke to you the other day, I didn't realize that you were the Chairman of a World Governing Body. Since your Board of Directors has seen fit to honor us by nominating their Chairman to work with us, the least we can do is reciprocate the honor. We would like you to be Chief Physician of our Team*".

It was, as you might imagine, awfully hard to remain blasé. I frankly nearly fell off my chair!

My longtime desire to go to the Olympic Games was to be realized, and not only as one of the team doctors for just any Country, but as Chief Physician for the greatest super power in Winter Sports….. and to that point only one or two DC's had even been to the Winter Games as Team DC's. It was really awesome.

One of the few people at that meeting was a man sitting quietly in a chair in the corner. If I told you that he was the prototype of everything we had always seen in the movies called "*spy*", it would be understatement. Dressed in a long black leather trenchcoat, black leather fedora, black tie, and black shoes… I conjured up the image of Boris Bad-enough from Rocky the squirrel. It was actually humorous in a stressed-out way. Minister Rusak told me, "*of course, you understand that you will need to be investigated by the KGB?*" I smiled broadly and answered, "*Really*?". He looked surprised at my smile, and said "*Why are you smiling?*"…. I replied "*I never thought of myself as important enough before to be investigated by the famous (I really wanted to say **in**famous) KGB*". The trenchcoat also smiled! Rusak said… "*you have said the right thing*!"… and then introduced me to the Colonel with [19]"*State security committee*".

Six Months before the Games….

I was now going to have to commit to being in Moscow every month for the six months leading up to the Games. And, I had business with the clinic anyway. So, that meant that I would have to go for two weeks per month for those months. The cost to me at home was staggering….. I later calculated it at around a $75,000 loss! And worth every penny.

---

[19] КГБ in Russian. It stands for State Security Committee or Государственный Комитет Безопасности

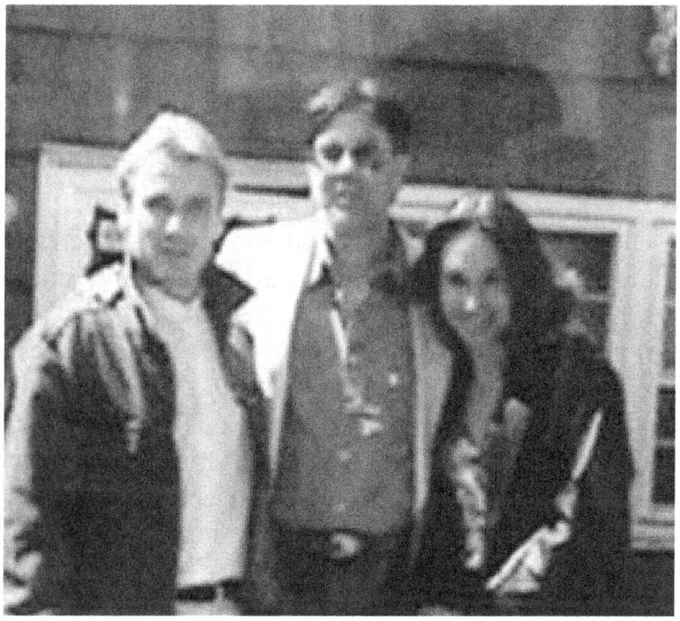

Fig 13 - Zhulin, the author and Usova

There were some really interesting events leading up to the actual event. Whenever I arrived in Moscow, I went to Sokolniki Stadium to see the skaters, and periodically to the Olympic Training Center at Novogorsk, not far from Sheremetyevo airport. The skaters were being coached at that time by Natalya Dubova, who, I think, saw an American doctor as something suspicious from the start. At that time, Maya Usova and Alexander Zhulin were not only skating partners but married as well. Sasha may not have been the model of a faithful husband it seems. In fact the whole group, because they were nearly always together, all beautiful people, and had spent their lives in this cloistered environment, was susceptible to a little round-robin hanky-panky.

The affairs

One day, Maya was crying on my shoulder that Sasha had been named in an interview by the mass media as having had an affair with Grishuk. It fell to me to console her, and I asked her how she knew it was true? She told me that not only had it been Grishuk who held a press conference to announce it, but that it hadn't been the first time either.... With whom was the first affair? That will have to remain a patient confidence, but suffice it to say.... appearances can be very deceiving! I told Maya that the fling with Grishuk was akin to the Nancy Kerrigan affair, only a kind of sexual Tonya Harding.. in that it looked like Grishuk had seduced Sasha (not too difficult it seems), precisely to come out to the world to accomplish exactly what nearly happened.... Maya was considering leaving Sasha. I told her if she did that, she would be giving Grishuk exactly what she wanted, and that she should just go out on that ice with her head held high and make believe that it was nothing to her at all.... and skate her heart out.

She did, and she and Sasha won a Bronze medal in Albertville, and went on to win a Silver in Lillehammer against Platov and Grishuk.... maybe it wasn't necessary? The scores in Lillehammer were one tenth of one point from one judge different.... Who knows?

Trust

Another time, I was videotaping the practice session and Sasha skated over to me and simply asked, "*you're not going to give that to the US Team are you*?"... I told him I would never violate my responsibility to them, inasmuch as they had entrusted me as their doctor to maintain their privacy. By the way, there is much more I could tell here, but the stories I have repeated are not based on patient confidentialities. And, I took my position and their trust very seriously indeed.

Unified Team

The REAL story behind what went on in Albertville is actually more interesting than at first glance. In the interim, i.e. between the time of my being appointed, and the Games, the Soviet Union disintegrates. But, there is not enough time for the now 15 separate Republics, which are almost independent Countries, to register individually as 15 National Olympic Teams. What to do? IOC President H.E., Juan Antonio Samaranch cuts a deal, in which the IOC agrees to allow the 15 Republics to call themselves "*Unified Team*" and march into the Olympic Stadium as though they were still one nation. But, there's no national flag, so we march under the flag of the IOC itself, and each athlete has to carry the flag of his or her individual Republic.

Naturally, the guy who was Zhuk's friend, was responsible for getting the credentials to the IOC in time for the games. This he , undoubtedly, deliberately failed to do for me. So, I arrived in Albertville full of expectation to work with the Soviet Team and find that my credential is no where to be found. The credentialing department has no mention of me on their list! In fact, they as much as tell me that I was "*fifth columned by my own team*". I run around trying to find the Chief of Mission for what is now called the "*Unified Team*".

He's hard to find, and time is running out to get a credential. Finally someone lets him know I'm here and he tells them to credential me as a guest! That means that I get no access to any of the Olympic Villages, and thus no access to my skaters to treat them! Emergency mode kicks in......

Mexico to the Rescue

They tell me at the credentialing agency that its now too late to get credentialed for village access, unless a member of the IOC Executive signs off on it. Luckily Mr Smirnov, is the IOC member from the USSR, and a vice-president of the

IOC. So, how to find him and then get him to sign off on this? I hit on a plan. I find the representative of Mexico's Olympic team, and he signs a paper authorizing me to be the Team Physician for Mexico as well. With this I can embarrass the Russian representative into credentialing me for the Unified Team, because he doesn't want me to be there for Mexico, while treating the Russian skaters and telling the news media about their dishonesty.

When Smirnov hears about the Mexican appointment, he signs off, and they credential me with Unified Team.

While in Albertville, the French Chiropractic Association hears that a DC is Chief Physician for the USSR, and since it was still [20]illegal in France to practice Chiropractic, they hold a "*Press*" conference, calling the entire Agence France Presse to the Press Centre in Albertville to hear Dr. Press press (oh well) his opinions about the French's choice in health care and my relationship with the Soviet Athletes.

Chiropractic in France

We get into the Press Centre, and they've prepared an interpreter and earphones for me to follow the French. I fail to wear them and they freak out.... But the fear turns to all smiles when I tell them in French that I don't need the earphones because I speak fluent French. I told them that they *"fought a revolution for 'Liberty, Fraternity and Equality', but you're not Libre (free)."* There's an audible *"huhhhh... "?* *"As long as you do not have free choice of health care. As long as the Ordre des Medicines holds a monopoly over your bodies, you cannot be truly free*". I got a standing ovation.

---

[20] Due to Napoleonic Code, any act not specifically made legal remains illegal, thus Chiropractic, as it is unregulated, remains an act only a medical doctor, untrained in it, may provide. At press time, there is a bill going through the French legislature to change this inequity.

Since the IOC had not yet provided any place where the athletes can get adjusted, the French Chiropractic Association kindly made arrangements for the owner of a hotel in Brides-les-Bains, where I was billeted, to provide a studio at street level for my use as a clinic. I was extremely grateful, until I received a bill in the mail after the games were over.

There were really very few injuries, and I actually worked very little at the Winter Olympics in treatment of athletes. Apparently we had done a good job preparing them for this event. I had been in Moscow every month for at least one week, to work with athletes for six months before the Games. It paid off, and I was able to enjoy the Games far more.

Defection

You may recall the run-in I had with the trainer at the US Olympic Training Center, Bob Beeten and his wife Jenny. While I was in Albertville, one afternoon at Brides-les-Bain, Wearing the Soviet Uniform, I ran into Jenny, who had to sarcastically ask me if I had "*defected?*". I just laughed and said, "*well, you didn't want my services, but the Soviet Union did... maybe they know something you don't?*"...

Brilliant English

Tanya and I were sitting in a small crêperie in Bride-les-Bain, when in walks a contingent of the US figure Skating team, including Christopher Bowman, and pals. Chris and I didn't know each other then, but I recognized him. Naturally, Tanya and I were talking in English and Russian, and I was dressed in a Soviet uniform... so when I turned to Chris Bowman and asked "*Hi Chris, how's the team doing*?" He seemed shocked.... Then I realized his surprise when he just stared at me, my uniform and Tanya for a full minute before saying "*You speak brilliant English*!"..... I laughed and said… "*thanks, five generations in the States will do that to you*!".

The CIA

Another evening early in the Games, we were at a nightclub, and there was a group of Americans talking at an adjacent table. Being the shy retiring type that I am, I chatted them up…. One guy tells us he's with the State Department. In the conversation, we're told that he's with the advance team for Vice-President Quayle who's making an appearance at the Games, and later that this fellow had previously been in North Korea, Cambodia and several other hot spots…. It was as close I guess, as he could come to just telling me he was a "*Company man*".

Remember at that point Tanya was just my girlfriend… and he took an instant liking to her… welllllll…. In any event, he was from that time all over her, and at one point, before we moved to a hotel, he had a French Gendarme officer knock on the door of the Soviet villa, and bring her two tickets to one of the prime events…. To her alarm, he even took her under some security fence to see another event….. so, we were now under scrutiny of the CIA as well…..

As I said, during the games I saw really very little of my skaters, Sasha Zhulin, Maya Usova, Evgeny Platov, Oksana Grishuk, and the others…before the games, in the preparation time it was another story. We were to become lifelong friends.

Judging corruption was rampant in figure skating. Everyone knew it was going on, but it was the dirty little secret that really no one saw fit to change until the Winter Games in Salt Lake City, which were already so tainted by the bribery scandal that kept Kim, Un Yong, a friend of Chiropractic's, from becoming President of the IOC, that it came as little surprise to anyone in the know when the Gold Medal in pairs was awarded to Elena Berezhnaya and Anton Sikharulidze, of where-else? Russia; and then due to the outcry, to the Canadians as well…! Actually, many judges I have spoken to, feel that the complexity of Elena and Anton's routine was SO much greater, that even with his stepping out of a turn, they actually deserved the Gold, despite the near perfect performance of the Canadians.

Tanya and I were sitting in Albertville at the skating venue, and we were watching the Dance competiton. The top seeded team was Natalia Klimova and Sergei Ponomarenko, of… Russia. The French team, brother and sister, Isabel and Paul DuChenais, were crowding the top. Sasha and Maya, were the favorites for the Silver and everyone assumed that Isabel and Paul would take Bronze. It was just like that then… reputation was very important.

Judging is bought

After Klimova and Ponomarenko skated, the scores were announced. Tanya and I were sitting about two rows behind Christopher Dean, who was at the time married to Isabel DuChenais, and most likely that's why he and Jane Torvill were not competing in Albertville…. I.e., so as not to take the opportunity from his bride. Anyway he was their coach too…. When the scores were announced …. (The technical merit scores are announced first and then artistic performance), there was such a wide margin left between the two groups of scores that anyone who knew the system was immediately and embarrassingly aware that the judges had deliberately left plenty of room for the DuChenais' to move into a higher place. So embarrassing was this overt favoritism that Chris Dean put his head in his hands in shame…. It was caught on camera.

There was then an intermission and we went across the street to the short track stadium and sat with Minister Rusak and a couple of his acolytes. Shortly the Russian Judge, who was working the Dance event, came over and said to Rusak in Russian, "*Sasha and Maya can't get the Silver*". Rusak demanded to know "*why?*"; "*Because the French have paid too much!*" I heard it, with my own ears! .... I was nauseous. I had really wanted to believe that at least at the Olympics, the judging was honest..... I walked out really depressed. Sasha and Maya got the Bronze, proving the point....

As we walked out, we were stopped by a Camera crew from a US National Television station who decided that Tanya and I were the best dressed couple around and we were interviewed on one of the US' networks... Tanya, ever the fashion plate, ate it up.

Special Advisor to Minister Partnov

Shortly after the Games, I was again in Moscow, and Tanya and I were in discussion with a Professor Yuri Partnov, who would become Minister of Sport and Tourism under Yeltsin. Partnov's daughter was interested in coming to America and I had the key... a scholarship to Chiropractic college... One evening over dinner, he suggests we might like to accompany him to the Kremlin! It was to be the celebration of the "*100 Days of Yeltsin's Presidency*" and there was going to be a big party... actually two parties, one for the regular invitees, and one for an "*inner circle*"... and we had tickets to the inner circle. On this occasion, I had my video camera, and took it along, never knowing if they'd let me in with it or not. When we arrived, dressed in our best finery, we were shown to seats in the great theatre and treated to a marvelous show. Afterwards Partnov shows us to a staircase and up several flights, and around a corner is a private banquet hall, where the dignitaries are all having "*zakuski*" (Hors d'oevres).

The "2nd Putsch" on Video

I was filming the activities, and noticed then Vice-President Alexander Rutskoi talking to a general. Tanya told me that he wasn't supposed to be friendly with this particular general for some reason or other. Mr. Ruslan Khasbulatov was there as well, and we had a brief conversation. Yeltsin was conspicuous by his absence, and it turns out that Rutskoi and Khasbulatov were the co-conspirators who were brewing a plot to take over the government.

While videoing that fateful plot, I was interrupted by presumably a KGB agent, who made me stop filming. It was absolutely amazing that they didn't confiscate the tape.

Before we knew it, Novy God (New Years) was coming. It was 1990, and about to be 1991, and it was still the Soviet Union.

Tanya and I heard about a party being organized at the Kremlin for the New Year's Eve celebration. Novy God, is the biggest Holiday in the Russian speaking world. And this would turn out to be the last celebration held in the Soviet held Kremlin.

Moscow is full of mysteries, and the Oktyabrskaya Hotel (now known as the Hotel Prezident) was no exception. Unknown even to most Muskovites, it was located in a closely guarded, walled compound next to the French Embassy. We got the name of the organizer from a mutual acquaintance, and ventured over to the Hotel Guard house, hoping that we could gain entrance. As had happened to me several times before, like in Geneva at the Soviet Consulate, I simply walked over to the guard on duty and in my unaccented Russian, appeared very officious and said only "*Dobre Vyecher*" (good evening)... the guard, apparently awed at the presence of so important looking a figure, and assuming me to be Russian, opened the gate. Once inside we approached the entrance of the Hotel, where we found the host of the party. He looked really shocked when I told him how I got in..... but we were quickly invited to join them that evening.... And what a party it was!

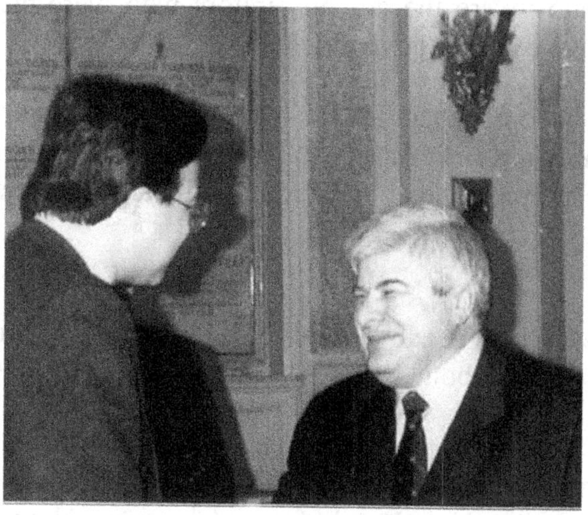

Fig 14 - the Author with the last Soviet Mayor of Moscow, Gavriil Popov in the Georgian Hall of the Kremlin

First there was a reception in the famous Georgian Hall. This is the regal Hall where the public had never been allowed before. It was the place that the Chairman of the Party would greet Heads of State, and Ambassadors presenting their credentials.

Everyone was there. Mayor Popov; The Archbishop of Moscow, presumably the 2nd in Command of the Russian Orthodox Church; Yakovlev, the Chairman of the Ostankino Broadcasting Company; people from Tass; every politician except Yeltsin and Gorbachev.... Yeltsin, probably too drunk that night like he was for his own party on the 100th day of his presidency, and only God knows what happened to Gorbachev that evening .... But everyone else was there. Actors, Actresses, and all the Russian social élite in all their finery.

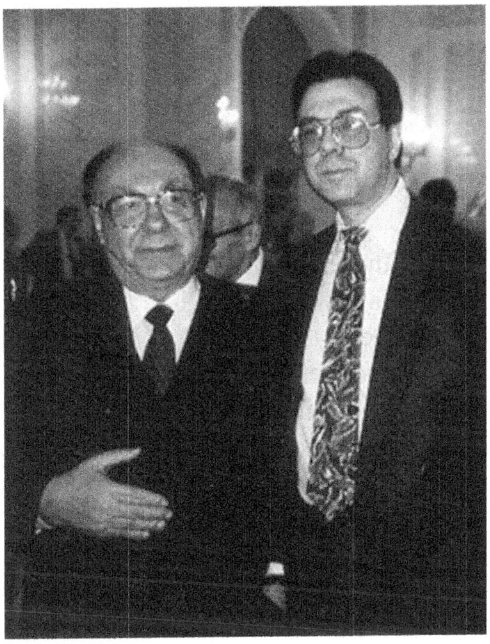

Fig 15 – With Yakovlev in the Georgian Hall

After cocktails and canapés in the Georgian Hall, we were given a tour of the Apartments of Ivan the Terrible. This too, was and still is off limits to the public. We then simply began wandering around on our own! No guards.... Again I thought I'm back in Petrodvoretz.... I started to open a door to a chamber, just to see what's inside when guards appeared and sharply stopped me. Then someone higher ranking apparently told them to stand down for us and I was allowed to enter.

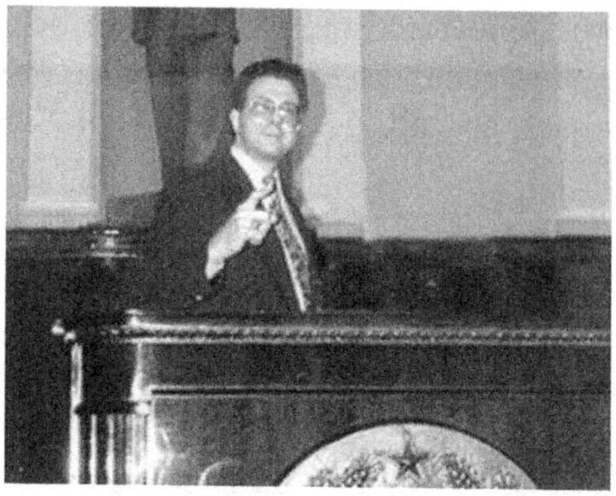

Fig 16 The Lenin Podium

I was standing in the Chamber of the Supreme Soviet. The first foreigner ever allowed in that hall! Tanya and I went up to the podium where Lenin gave his fiery addresses and stood with his statue behind me at his podium and posed with one hand in a pointing position like his official portrait and the statue were posed. Tanya's friend Lena had also finagled a ticket to the shindig as our mutual friend Alexei Kucherenko was then a student and journalist and took her as his date. She tried to photograph us standing there, but framed the picture too close to really see the position of us in true reference…. I wouldn't know it until I returned home to New Jersey.

When we were shown into the banquet hall for dinner, a fireworks display began which has diminished all subsequent displays for me, as the rockets shot from the Kremlin walls towards the Russian sky, I was filled with awe and wonder at the circumstances which brought a Jewish Doctor from the Bronx to his apogee professionally. I could only imagine what my ancestors who fled the Russian pogroms, would have thought about their descendant standing in the midst of such magnificence and in the seat of Soviet power.

Just when I thought it couldn't get better, the food came out and seemed to never stop as we were regaled with the finest cuisine that the Russian government could afford to provide... it was a banquet fit for the Czar. Just then the Soviet Army Chorus filed onto the stage and began to sing. One beautiful piece of Russian music after another until their finale.... It was announced... could I believe my ears? They would, in honor of their American guests, sing, in English, "*God Bless America*".... No! Had the Soviet Union come to this? Tanya was furious at what she saw as their kowtowing to our financial contributions to their economy.... I on the other hand was moved to real tears....

I guess America had a greater impact on the Soviet world than we imagined.... And we would only have to wait a few months to see the West's goal come to fruition as the entire Soviet Union collapsed around us.

People were at the same time scared and elated. Afraid the regime would come back, and afraid that it wouldn't. After all, they had obtained freedom, of sorts. But with freedom comes responsibility to your country and to your society. What the Russians got for some ten years was what they were qualified for, anarchy.

Like Lincoln freeing the slaves, the Russian people who had suffered the bloodiest history in the World were free to leave, to build businesses, and so on... after 800 years of one bloody ruler after another.

This was a highly literate lot of slaves, and these people had known a black market system that was the only way to get anywhere, or have anything. So anyone who did, was automatically corrupt in their genre. But it was the de facto means of functioning in their society. Were there people who were truly honest? Real Communists who really tried to "*build communism*"... sure... But I really believe that the vast majority were "*radishes*", i.e. red on the outside and white on the inside.

Chapter 15

After the Ball is Over

**

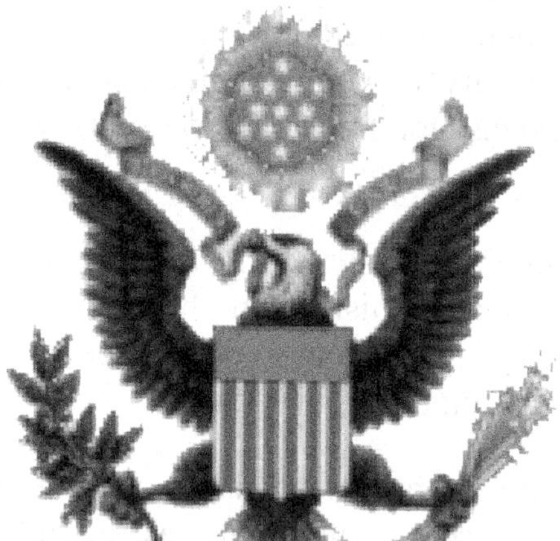

After the Olympic Games, my career, one would have thought, would really take off. The average person would assume that having been Chief Physician at the Olympics would be really great for my practice.

It would prove to be an asset, but there were still no lines waiting for me.. In fact, all the time I spent away from the office, during all that time, cost me a lot of patients. People just got tired of waiting for me to come home from my numerous trips and went elsewhere, even if they really thought I was better. At least they thought, this one's around.

Still, it did bring new patients and I continued to operate a reasonably profitable practice. In the professional sphere however, I continued to garner recognition and ever greater positions in the administrative/political world in sports medicine. And, anytime I wanted into something, doors seemed to open now that had been shut just a few months earlier.

Expert Testimony/Flying Donkeys

A rotund lady was shopping in a supermarket in Hudson County, NJ and fell on a banana peel. Sounds like a cartoon right? No, it really happened that way. Anyway, she goes to a Chiropractor and is diagnosed with three herniated discs and treated reasonably there. After some six to eight months of therapy her Doctor is called to a deposition at the office of the Defense Counsel.

After the preliminaries are over, he starts asking the standard questions of the Doctor. Then he asks, "*Doctor, have you ever had your license suspended or revoked anywhere?*". Doctor X answers "*Yes*". Oops… the patient's case is apparently over here…. He's asked what was the cause? He apparently did a year in Lewisberg Federal Penitentiary for manufacturing fictitious patients and billing for their treatment in cahoots with a lawyer who also did time for this Federal mail and insurance fraud.

Desperate, the Plaintiff's lawyer calls me to see if I can help. After examining the files and history, and doing my own physical on the patient, I come to the conclusion that her injuries are in fact from a fall like she describes and consistent with the time frame in which she allegedly fell. I agree to testify. Naturally, I cannot base my opinion on anything this felon-Doctor wrote or said, or his history can be brought into the trial testimony.

The case comes to Court, and the supermarket doesn't even retain another Chiropractor to testify against me. They hire instead, the chief of Orthopedics from a major local hospital, hoping to impress the jury against my testimony and help their Client avoid having to pay damages. They didn't count on my repartee in Court. The actual trial went something like this:

They bring in their big medical gun. It takes a half hour to have him qualified as an expert witness and tell the jury that a. the MRI was not of diagnostic quality and b. the injuries were due to normal aging, not a fall. I am brought in and they take nearly an hour to go over my credentials and get me accepted as an expert witness, to the detriment of the Defense side.

Finally defense Counsel, we'll call him Mr K starts questioning me….

Mr. K - Dr. Press, if I were to tell you that Dr X, an Orthopedic Surgeon, Chief of Orthopedics at XYZ Hospital has just testified, and he told the jury that this was not the result of an injury at all, but the normal result of aging, would that be of interest to you?

Me - Not at all.

Mr K -No? Tell me Doctor Press, why not?

Me - Well, you went to great lengths to brag about the qualifications of Dr. X, and we understand that he's an Orthopedic Surgeon.... Right?

Mr. K -Right

Me - Then, let's understand that I was qualified as an Expert in Chiropractic... I was Chief Physician of the Soviet Olympic Team, Chairman of the World Governing Body for my specialty, and all....So.... When a patient comes to me, it's my job to determine of he or she is a Chiropractic patient, or requires referral to a surgeon or other practitioner. Once I have determined that the patient is a Chiropractic case, as I did in the case of Mrs Y, the opinions of an Orthopedic surgeon are no longer of any interest to me whatsoever.

Mr. K Ok, Dr. then suppose we take a hypothetical situation, ok?

Me- Ok

Mr. K Dr. Press, suppose Mrs Y were to present in your office with this situation, and it was not from a fall at all, but....

Me- Counselor, let me interrupt you... let me get this straight... you're asking me if we were to graft wings onto a jackass, could it fly? (jury is laughing).

Mr K- Now Doctor, let's stay away from the Jackass and the wings, etc... you were qualified as an expert in Chiropractic, not Veterinary surgery, ok?

Me- Counselor... was Dr. X qualified in Veterinary surgery? Because it seems to have been he who put the wings on the Jackass! (jury is raucously laughing now).

Mk K- Your Honor, may we take a short break?

The supermarket settles…. Profitably.

Herb Perez

One day I was reading the paper, and heard that a guy I had met by coincidence in a restaurant in Fort Lee because I started a conversation over his USOC jacket, had just been named coach of the World team for the World Championships of Tae Kwon Do. Herb Perez was the only man to win a gold medal at the Olympics in Seoul in Tae Kwon Do, from the US. The article said the team was training at his Do Jang in nearby Cliffside Park. I drove over there the same afternoon, and found him receptive to having me work with the team. It seems the US Tae Kwon Do Federation had named four team docs, and none of them had offered to see the athletes before the actual competition. So, it was a great relief to have a team doc actually see them every day for a couple of weeks before the event. He got me credentialed, and I went to New York as US Team Doctor, 1993.

Soon I would receive a call from my old friend Dr. Luis Valera. Luis was a team doctor for Venezuela in the 1984 Olympics in Los Angeles. A friend at that time of Leroy Perry, he was invited through Perry to participate, and used his family connections to the then President of Venezuela to obtain the appointment.

Off to Caracas

Luis was President of the Venezuelan Chiropractic Association, and became an early member of FICS, so we were always rather good friends. Luis was from a really well to do family in Venezuela. I think I heard that his father owned his own airline. Luis' call was to invite me to Caracas, as President of FICS, together with a couple of our people. Drs Stephen Perle; now a professor at the University of Bridgeport's Chiropractic College, and a doctor Greene; who was a young DC traveling around South America at the time, who presumably knew the culture. We were to come to Caracas, as guests of President Perez, to lecture at the Venezuelan pentagon, before all the medical corps of the Venezuelan Military, and before the Medical staff of the Venezuelan National Oil Company, Maraven.

When the Venezuelan Airlines plane arrived in Caracas, there was an announcement over the loudspeaker..."*will all passengers please remain seated, as the government has requested, as a military escort is boarding to greet a dignitary*". I never dreamed it was for me.... But there was the escort, in full military regalia, a Colonel no less, aide to the Chairman of the Venezuelan Joint Chiefs of Staff, General of Quatro Soles, (four suns) Generalissimo Lara. A customized bulletproof van drove us straight to the pentagon... we didn't even pass through customs or immigration! That is real power.

For several days our every need was seen to by the Colonel, who offered and showed us delights which my married status at that time made it impossible to accept, and difficult to refuse without causing insult.

Eating Rat

One afternoon, we were told that there would be a state luncheon in my honor, and we were driven to the banquet hall for a meeting with General Lara, and General Maya, another very high ranking Officer. Only when seated, I was asked if I ever had tasted "*llapa*" ? I inquired what it was, and was told "*Capybara*". My colleagues in turn asked me what we were eating, and I just said, "*I'll tell you later.*

Enjoy it, it's really good'. I really wanted to avoid an incident, should either of them have a problem consuming the world's largest rodent. It was served in a raspberry sauce and really was delicious.

By the time our sojourn in Caracas was ending, I was sorely tempted to emigrate to Venezuela.

I no sooner got back to the States, then another call, this time from Dr. Stoxen in Illinois, suggested that I go to England to work the World Arm Wrestling Championships, in Kent. It sounded like another adventure, so I accepted and took off for merry olde England again.

Black Lion Sport Center

Arriving at the Black Lion Sport Centre, I set up shop and was greeted warmly by the meet director. During the second day, a representative of the Swiss National team came to me for help.... It seems that one of their number was entrusted with the safekeeping of a quantity of watches with the logo of the Swiss Arm Wrestling Federation imprinted on the faces, as well as a cache of camera gear belonging to the members of the team. He was told not to let it out of his sight for a second and still put it down somewhere. In an instant it was "*nicked*" (stolen).

Kent Constabulary

None of the team spoke English , and only one spoke French fairly well, as they were a German Canton, so they needed my help to call the Police. I got on the telephone, and reached the local Constabulary, whereupon a "*Bobby*" was dispatched. When he got to the Sport Centre, I translated the story of the Swiss team to him and he determined that being an international event, he needed higher authority as back-up. Soon the Chief Inspector of the Kent Constabulary appeared. I identified myself, both as medical director, and as a speaker of French, as well as showing him my shield as ex-Chief of Auxiliary Police, and he asked if I could translate the complaint in both English and French. When I told him my French was good enough for that, he actually asked the Swiss Captain too, and was told my French was "*better than mine*".

When I finished this lengthy task, the Chief inspector turned to the Bobby and said, "I think our brother officer deserves something special don't you?'... the Bobby said "yes sir..." and started to take off his badge! I told them I couldn't accept his badge... but the Bobby told me that the numbers are snap in plastic and he can get another as soon as he returns to the station. We all went back to the Constabulary for a pint... yes, they actually have their own pubs at the Constabularies. Actually this is very clever.. for several reasons....

Firstly, it keeps the police at home, i.e. at the Constabulary in the evenings, as it gives them a hang-out; and,

Secondly, it provides a way to keep any drunken behavior hidden from the public; and,

Thirdly, it allows for the rapid mobilization of men to a crime scene should strong back-up be required.... I think it's brilliant.

They inducted me into the Kent Constabulary as an honorary member, and presented me the classical helmet of a Bobby in addition to the Badge. It was spring and I was in a suit jacket. The Chief inspector told me to hide the helmet, because everyone will want one as this is "*the*" trophy of England, he said. I just started laughing.... How to hide it? If I put it under my jacket, I'd look like Dolly Parton after a mastectomy! When I said this, the whole lot caught my laughter and it broke up the whole station house for ten minutes.

Skating Rolls Back Into My Life

In my skating career, I have enjoyed a love-hate relationship with the sport. I loved to skate, and hated the politics in it. When I began my professional career, and was back in New Jersey from Iowa, I went to skate at Paramus Skating Rink. Andy and Mary were long gone, and the rink had no pro to speak of at the time, so I approached the owner Gus Camerano, to see if I could take on a class. I frankly figured it might be good for me to develop patients too. Naturally, Gus made it clear from the start that he didn't want me soliciting anyone as a patient… remember, in those days many people thought Chiropractors were tantamount to witchdoctors, and he didn't want to endorse that in his precious rink…..still we agreed on a program.

I taught a class for a while, and Gus and I parted company due to the rink getting ready to close. Today it's a window treatment and a pet shop. So, I started to go back to Montvale Rink, which was a little further away from me. But, I was friendly with Phil Pinto, the pro there, having taken lessons from him for some years.

First Aid Fiasco

On several occasions someone would get injured in my presence, and being trained not only as a physician, but long before as an EMT, I ran to provide first aid. All seemed ok, until one day, a boy fell during a matinee session and broke his arm. The fracture was an open fracture and was bleeding from an artery. I immobilized the fracture in place, stopped the bleeding, treated him for shock, and held pressure until the ambulance arrived. Then the owner, Lou Colicchio, came over to me…. "*you have to stop doing this*", he said. I was incredulous… "*what are you talking about*?" I demanded. "*Treating people in my rink*", he stammered. I just looked at him and thought "*what an ass!"*…. but said, "*Lou, I'm providing first aid as a good Samaritan, not treating people*". He went on, "*welllll, we really have to leave this to the professionals, cause I could be sued, if you make a mistake*".

I foolishly continued to argue. And arguing with fools is always foolish. I went on… "*Lou, I'm a physician, licensed to practice in New Jersey. What kind of professionals are you talking about?*" He said "*the Ambulance people*". I told him…"*the ambulance people are EMT-s, of which I am also an EMT, and I taught EMT's for the State... moreover they have just 125 hours of training to become EMT's and as a physician, I have over 5000!*" …. But as fools will, he continued… "*still, they are the ones paid to do this, and you're just volunteering*"… I can't believe that I took the trouble to actually answer this last stupidity…. "*Lou*", I tried, "*they are the Volunteer Ambulance Corps... that means that they are Volunteering too....*" Having nothing of any sense to counter with, he just said, "*well, you have to decide... you can continue to skate here if you stop doing that.*" I said, Lou, there's a good Samaritan law, which says that "*no one who renders emergency treatment in good faith may be held in civil damages, except for acts of omission or acts of commission.... That means that as a licensed physician, if I stand by and deliberately do nothing while someone bleeds to death, which is apparently what you would prefer, THEN I can be sued and you would probably go to jail for interfering with my attempt to help....*" He just looked at me and said…. "*well then you can't skate here anymore.*" I left and told him…. "*Lou, you're a real jerk... one day you'll die or sell, and THEN I'll come back*"…..

Well he finally did sell to a really bright and pleasant guy, Bob Dill, and now I skate there again, and help all those injured when I'm around.. Only I lost a lot of my skating skills from the 15 years Collichio's stupidity cost me.

Research

About the same period, about 1979, I was deeply involved in research in skating biomechanics and its relationship to Chiropractic. I even went into debt to buy what was then the only real option in video gear, a professional ¾" setup with a camera and "*luggable*" deck etc. I took it to several club sessions around the state, and taped practices and skater/volunteers to measure their limb length and weight balance, and see them skate forwards and backwards inside and outside edges.

Roller Skating Rejects Research

After a while I became convinced that I had enough data to write it up, and could predict the outcome of a competition, in dance skating, if I first measured the skaters' leg lengths and their weight imbalances on twin scales. One could graph their averaged measurements and place them on a scale. They would win in order of their measurements! I took it to Nationals, got a bunch of skaters to volunteer and actually called the outcome to within 95% accuracy. Naturally, the powers that were, refused to let me do this officially and when I submitted my paper, a guy who was their Executive Director actually overrode the editor of their magazine, refusing my publication, saying instead that "*it's just from some Chiropractor. He's probably just trying to promote himself.*" Another jerk! MD's were serious researchers, and only doing it altruistically, but DC's were just self-promoting??? Who decided that? So, I just submitted my paper to the Professional Skater's Guild of America and they happily published this pioneering work in sports medicine.

Plagiarism

I later got another unhappy surprise form my own sport, when the USARS appointed a California podiatrist to the position of US National Team Doctor, and in what seemed his first official act, he essentially stole my paper, publishing nearly the same data as though he did the research, just a couple of months later!

FIRS Vindicates me

Considering my past with the Roller Skating association, the next bit of history would be a real pleasure.... Some twenty years later, in the afternoon, I was taking a break from my work, and was feeling a bit bored. So, I went online, and for whatever reason was in my head at the moment, I thought to take a look at the web-site for the World Governing Body of Roller Sports, known as Fédération Internationale de Roller Skating or FIRS. This was my sport after all and early in my career, their American branch, known as a National Governing Body (NGB) had snubbed me, when I tried to get them to publish my work on weight balance in skaters. In fact it was the ice skating association which happily took brought my research to their membership, not my own sport. I was depressed and hurt.

Finding a nice webpage for FIRS, I started through it looking for a medical commission, and lo and behold, at first scan, found no mention of one there. So, I checked the officers and found an e-mail for the President, Sr. Isidro Oliveras in Barcelona, and sent him a note saying that this was my own sport, that I had been with the USSR Olympic team, etc., and if he wanted a medical commission, I was available to work with him.

Then I went back to the website and went through it again. Oh no! This time I saw a reference to a medical doctor from Portugal, listed as their medical commission chairman... I quickly sent a second e-mail.... "*oops*" I said. "*I found the doctor's name , but if you would like me to work with him, I would do that too*".

By a miracle of coincidence, I got an e-mail back in a couple of days, from Sr. Oliveras himself, saying that although Dr. X was listed there, that "*since his appointment some seven years previous, they had never heard from him at all, in all that time*", and he was interested in talking to me... he was "*coming to New York in a couple of weeks, would I be available to meet?*"

When we met at his hotel in the big apple, Sr. Oliveras was an aristocratic, gracious host, and a pleasure to talk to. The upshot of that meeting was that he wanted me to be President of a real Medical Commission and bring them into the twentieth century. I was elated.... Vindication at last!

I spent the next two years, part time of course, in addition to my practice duties, working diligently for the betterment of the skaters of the world. FIRS had some 55 National Associations, and was an IF, i.e. International Federation, which meant that it was the recognized World Governing Body for all Roller Sports. Recognized by whom? By the International Olympic Committee (IOC), and the General Association of International Sports Federations (GAISF), and other agencies. No other Chiropractor had ever even been an ordinary member of the medical commission of an IOC recognized IF before... And, there were only about 75 sports recognized, so this meant that there were only about 300 physicians worldwide in this position, and I was now one of that elite cadre of only about 75 Presidents. OK, roller sports are not yet in the Olympic Games, and it would have been even a greater achievement had I been on one of the actual Olympic sport's IF's medcoms, but this is still a huge honor, and a breakthrough first for my profession.

Treachery in Australia

The party lasted only about two years though. In developing the protocol for Roller Sports to have an Anti-Doping Code, I ran headlong into opposition from the two MD's appointed to work under my leadership. Strangely, it was due to my insistence on following the spirit and letter of the IOC Anti-Doping Code. The US Team Doctor, it seems, wanted to be able to hand out beta-agonist inhalers, the type given to sufferers of asthma, at a competitive venue, even after the competition had begun.

These inhalers are considered a banned substance unless the athlete actually has exercise induced asthma. Also they have anabolic steroid-like effects given over time. The IOC had a policy which made it clear this was tantamount to cheating, if the athlete was not really a asthma sufferer, but merely one having trouble with endurance at altitude for example. Yet this was precisely what he wanted to do.

The FIRS Coup

I tried to reason with him. Explaining that this thinking was perhaps expected of the National team Doctor, but that as a member of the IF Medical Commission, we had to have rules preventing just one team from what was really a form of cheating. He was not deterred. Instead, he got together with his friend, a lady MD from Australia, and together they undermined my authority at a Board meeting in Australia where I would have had to pay my own way to attend. While I was not looking they got their NGB's to form a coalition and outvoted President Oliveras, and got me replaced with one of their own, to get their way. Frankly, I think I was set up..... It was perhaps not for the inhalers at all, that they pulled this coup, but just to be rid of the Chiropractor who was their boss.

Kirsan and Aleks

I really didn't care too much anyway, because just as this was all starting to brew, I got a call from one of Tanya's classmates from Moscow, Alexei Kucherenko. Alexei it seems had done quite well for himself since the days when I visited him at the obshchyezhit (dormitory) at GiMO the Institute for Foreign Relations. While at school, Aleks became friendly with a character named Kirsan Ilyumzhinov. Both were geniuses and brilliant linguists. Aleks in Hungarian, and Kirsan in Japanese.

Kirsan was from a little known region of Russia, called Kalmykia. Bordering on the Caspian, just across from Iran, it's the only Tibetan Buddhist region in the former USSR. They have their own language (nearly extinct but being resurrected), and culture too, having been descended from the Mongols.

Kirsan, on graduation, returned to Elista, the Kalmykian capital and got himself elected President of Kalmykia... going to Japan, he finagled a deal with some Japanese bankers to open a bank in Elista, if he could get the Russian Duma (Parliament) to enact a law giving tax free zone status to Kalmykia. Presumably the Duma figured collectively that no one would want to go to Kalmykia anyway, and the taxfree status wouldn't help much. They were wrong! Kirsan got the status, and the bank and used the position to buy up every voucher that was issued to Kalmykian workers when the USSR privatized whatever industry was in Kalmykia. And they had enough, like Caviar and Sturgeon harvesting facilities and oil, that Kirsan, in just ten years became one of the richest men in the World. Thirty-six years old and a multi-Billionaire!

Aleks too following whatever Kirsan told him, invested everything, and also became super-wealthy, though not on the same scale... perhaps a few zeros less....?? Aleks had become the Chief of the Administration of the Republic of Kalmykia, a diplomat, and a wheeler-dealer.

Kirsan, as President of a semi-autonomous Republic and member of the upper house of the Duma was now wielding much power in Russia. Enough to be considered one of the

"*Oligarchs*", ruling the Country. This placed him in constant personal and physical danger. Naturally no one outside of Russia has heard of Kalmykia, so who would care if he got knocked off? So, what to do? Kirsan plays Chess. He gets involved in the politics of the World Governing Body of Chess, and by putting near $50,000,000.00 , that's Fifty MILLION dollars in play, gets himself elected to the Presidency of the Chess World Governing Body too, known as FIDE. Now an international public figure, he feels a little more secure about his stature and at least figures that if someone tries to kill him, they'll know that it will make news everywhere. Clever man!

Chess, however, is still not a part of the Olympic Games.... So Kirsan commissions a panel to create a white paper to submit to the IOC and get Chess recognized as a sport. He goes straight to the IOC, bypassing all the traditional routes to IOC recognition, and by adroitly lobbying the members, gets it.... Chess is a sport.

When Aleks first told me this, I warned him that FIDE would now need a Medical Commission and that they would have to comply with the IOC Anti-Doping Statutes. He laughed... "*Chess? No?*" I told him it was true, and that it would be just a matter of time before they are ordered to do this. He told Kirsan who also laughed....

Jay Leno's Monologue

Just about the time that my MD cohorts in FIRS were planning their coup, the IOC was telling Kirsan that he needed a Medical Commission, and an anti-doping plan. This was to be a huge undertaking, because every other sport already knew that it was a sport, and everyone was prepared to participate in this. Chess players, on the other hand, had no inkling that they were athletes and never dreamed that someone would come along and demand a sample of their pee, never mind to test it for steroids.... The whole world laughed.... Jay Leno even did a monologue one evening about my work, as I was in Massachusetts telling the US Chess Federation that they would have to conform. But, just as FIRS decided that I had served my mandate, FIDE called to offer me to run their Medical Commission, though as Vice-President, not President.

They were so apologetic about that too..... I was told that unfortunately they had a clause in their Statutes which required that if there was someone qualified on their Presidential Board, that a Chairmanship had to go to him/her. And, there was a pediatric anesthesiologist on their Board, from El Salvador. Moreover, I was told that Dr. Pedro Barrera was a member of the El Salvadoran Parliament, and President of the Pan American Chess Federation, and thus was so busy that I would be in virtual charge of the Commission, and free to run it as I saw fit.

I accepted the position. Moreover, it was clear that for the first time I would be given enough compensation for my time away from the office, that it would be profitable for me to do this. Previously, in FIRS, also for the first time, I was actually compensated for my expenses.... Remember, Chiropractors were interested in doing these things, not only for the altruistic effect on sport, but also because it was a feather in the collective caps of the profession, and as an after effect, it could boost ones credibility at home and thus increase ones practice. Not an unreasonable expectation for a volunteer doctor taking his time away from his office....

But this time, it would actually become profitable.... I was promised full business class airfare, even if I flew coach.... I was promised a per diem for hotels and a per diem for meals, plus reimbursement for all FIDE related expenses too, and $300/day for every day I was out of the office, or $900.00/week.... Thus, if I went somewhere for a two week stint, and flew coach, and stayed in 2 or 3 star hotels, I could come back with 5-6 thousand over my expenses and that meant I could do this for a living. I was thrilled. I would have happily done this instead of Chiropractic practice.

Naturally, the first time I spoke to Barerra, and he heard there was a Chiropractor who was supposed to run things, he told me that he "*planned to be a very hands on Chairman*"... so much for promises!

The relationship with Barerra was rocky from the start, but they needed my expertise, and he knew that he didn't know this stuff.... So, after all I was able to work my way through the political maze for a while..... when he figured he knew enough to live without me, he started to plot to get rid of me.

I smelled a rat, and started to tape our conversations. He fully okayed all the policy I suggested. Especially the financial reimbursement recommendations I implemented. I was even told by Mrs. Barrera how much she liked me, because he "*had never seen nickel one from FIDE before, paying everything out of his own pocket"*. And, now he would get paid for this Medical Commission stuff...

So, when we went to Mendoza, Argentina for the PanAm Youth Chess Championships, he was setting me up to accuse me of taking more than I was spending.... At least he tried. I had accounted for every penny. So that didn't work.... He still needed a way to oust the Chiropractor.... So, when we got to Halkidiki, in Macedonia, just before the 9/11 disaster, he got a representative of the US Chess Federation to make a motion that no one but the President should get Business fare... this took several thousands for each trip out of my pocket and thus made it impracticable for me to continue to travel for the federation. They also made a motion to have us do as much as possible through local representatives instead of actually going to venues ourselves, and that made travel nearly impossible.... I just stopped working for them. Eventually, Barrera died suddenly and they quietly replaced me.

The 9/11 affair

Just before 9/11 I was in Macedonia, in my capacity as Vice-President of the FIDE (Chess Federation) Medical Commission. I left for home that night of 9/10 and arrived in Vienna in time to leave for the USA about 10:00 AM i.e., 4:00PM 9/10 NY time. We had traversed nearly the whole Atlantic when the Chief Cabin Steward came to me for help.

Usually, I identify myself to the cabin people on check –in as Doctor, and tell them that I speak several languages and will be available in emergency. This was an emergency. I was told only that "*a gentleman in coach* (thank God I was in Business Class, courtesy of FIDE) *had chest pains*". It seems they didn't have any Russian speakers in the crew, and the entire coach section was filled with Byelorussians emigrating to the US from Minsk.

I checked the man out and ascertained that his pain was likely from indigestion, as it immediately subsided after I gave him some antacid tablets. So, I said "*it's ok, we can go on to New York*". By that point the Chief cabin steward came over and said ominously, "*the Captain wants to see you*". I went at once to the cockpit. The usually affable Captain had a dour look on his face and said… "*that's the problem, we can't go on to the US*". I said "*huh*?" He continued, "*We just got a news report that the entire North American airspace is closed. The US is under attack. The financial district of New York is in ruins, the pentagon has been hit and I don't know if world War three has begun or what… and we can't land anywhere on the continent. We are ordered to return to Europe*". I gulped and said.. "*do we have enough gas?*" he said "*just*".. Just? So, I inquired, "*where are we going to land*?". He said "*London*". Some five hours later… it was now about 9:30PM London time, i.e. 2:30AM, New York time, already 9/12 there!

We were approaching London, when the Captain called me back.... He said... "*Doc, we have another problem*".... "*What?*" I asked... he said, "*Tony Blair has just closed off London airspace too, and we can't land there either!* " Now really scared, I inquired... "*is there enough fuel for that?*"... now he just said "*I hope so*"... I swallowed hard.... I listened as he called the Manchester tower... "*Manchester tower... this is Austrian Air flight ###, heavy, requesting clearance to land*".... After what seemed a long time... I heard these words I shall never forget... "*in that case Manchester tower, I am declaring a fuel emergency, and we are landing, unless you plan to blow us out of the sky*". Now I held my breath for what seemed like half an hour.... In reality it was probably a couple of minutes.... When he said... "*Thank you Manchester for the clearance*".... Now it was just a question of whether we would run out of fuel as we were landing, or glide into town without engines... we made it of course.

They kept us on board while we re-fueled. Presumably afraid someone would escape into England. We were still to return that night to Vienna. And arrived at 2:00AM Vienna Time... on 9/12. We had been in transit for some 16 hours!

I must say that Austrian Air and the Austrian people were marvelous to us. We were put up at a five star hotel, and all meals were taken care of. On arrival, we were shown, coach business and first class, all, to the first class lounge, with a large staff on hand in the middle of the night to help us... they handed us cell phones and told us that for the duration of our stay, all calls would be free to anyone, as frequently as we needed to call, to anywhere on Earth.

At 8:00AM that same morning there was a meeting and we were told that they didn't know how long we would be marooned in Europe, but they assumed it would be at least Saturday or Sunday before we could go home.

I approached the manager and bargained… Saying… "*you're going to pay for our hotel and meals while here ? So, why not give me a round trip business class ticket to Basle in Switzerland, and I can come back when you are ready to ship us out*". He inquired "*what was better in Basle"*?. I told him I spoke rather bad German and even less Wiener Deutch, He reminded that in Basle they too speak German, and an even more difficult version… I told him… "*but Basle is on the border, with Mulhouse, France and I speak fluent French, and anyway had a girlfriend near Mulhouse*". They agreed, and I spent the time at Pascale's place.

Chapter 16

Practicing Chiropractic in America

**

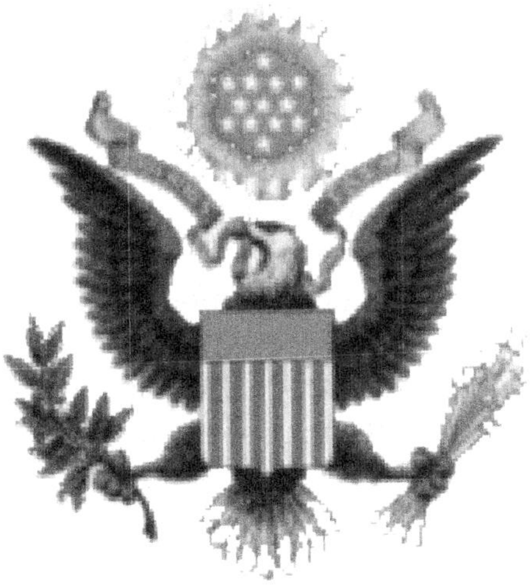

About the time the work with FIDE was starting, the laws in New Jersey and Nationally too, were changing regarding insurance coverage. It would alter my life in ways I could not imagine.

Starting around 1997 I was treating many patients who had been in auto accidents. Despite that people had real injuries, frequently they didn't even really know it, but knew that they could make money in a lawsuit, and sought legal counsel. So many times it was a lawyer who told them to see a Chiropractor. To be honest, though for the wrong motives, it was clear that these people had actually suffered whiplash injuries, and if not sent by their lawyers, they may not have known about their injuries for three to five years, when their discs would degenerate to the point that they would develop pain and spasm. Then it would require far more treatment to fix it, and the problem would become chronic.

The Right Thing for the Wrong Reason

So they were doing the right thing for the wrong reason. As a physician, I was obligated to treat them when I found a real injury, whether anyone would believe that they were injured or not, if I, in my own mind as a doctor knew that they were hurt I HAVE to treat them. Unfortunately, the insurance carriers also figured out that people were not hurting when they presented for treatment, and this they conveniently equated with fraud on the part of the patients. Did they care if these people had actually suffered real injuries? Absolutely not! Did they care what was the result of ignoring these problems? Absolutely not! Did they even believe that there were real injuries? Also no.... thus the Chiropractic profession was in the awful position of being the profession already a little suspect, taking this unpopular position that injuries people themselves may not have known they had were necessary to treat, and worse yet, that the carriers should be forced to pay for that.

Hospital Privileges

One afternoon, I get a call from out of the blue. Who is it? Dr. William Cirino, Sr., DC, the former member of the Board of Medical Examiners from when I took my license exam, and father of one of my classmates at New York. He is soliciting my assistance in writing some paperwork for Preakness Hospital, and offers me staff privileges if I help him. I guess, my reputation is really getting around! Naturally, I offer to help the man, and over the ensuing several years Bill and I become close friends. In fact he becomes a surrogate father to me in some ways.

Interesting cases

Early in my career, after taking a course in Applied Kinesiology, I came back to my office and was teaching a class in CPR. One of the students came on crutches. We started a conversation, and I soon discovered that she was an RN with a Master's in Nursing. We'll call her Cathy. Cathy was 32 years old at that time, and I was told that in addition to her low back pain, she was numb from the knee down in her left leg.

Cathy had already suffered 2 myocardial infarctions (heart attacks) and was diagnosed with a condition known as Systemic Lupus Erythematosus, or SLE. In this condition, the body turns on itself, and starts to develop antibodies to its own tissues, progressively attacking one organ system after another, eventually killing the victim. In Cathy's case, the disease had already attacked her heart, thus the attacks, her kidneys, liver and other places. Due to the high levels of Steroids they had her take, she had developed the classical "*moon face*" and "*buffalo hump*", and put on serious weight. She already had two total hip replacement operations due to the softening effects of the Steroids on her bones, and was developing osteoporosis in her proximal tibia (the top of her lower leg).

The Doctors had given her six months to live. Still, she was intent on fighting this disease, and was taking a CPR class, ostensibly to get her mind off her troubles.

She came to the office to see me, skeptical that I could do anything for her, but trying just this last thing to make her more comfortable. Initially it was just her back pain that motivated her to try Chiropractic. But while lying on my table, I got the bright idea that the osteoporosis in her leg was due to disuse, not the disease. That is, she was using crutches and not putting her weight on the leg. Moreover, I started putting finger pressure on acupoint (similar to acupuncture, except without needles) sites in her foot, and while squeezing one of them she cried out.... "*ouch*!"... I asked "*ouch what*?" She said *"my foot hurts, you're hurting me*". Then, "*Oh my God, I FEEL my left foot*!".... she walked out of the office without her crutch, much to the utter amazement of her waiting family.

Then she asked me what I could do for the Lupus? I told her that I cannot hold out a hope of cure for an auto-immune disease, but at least we could attack the problems of what is wrong with her homeostasis (natural chemical balance). I considered what could be at the origin of this aberration of normal cells that cause them to attack one's own body? Then I realized that stress can diminish the adrenal gland output so much that the body's own anti-inflammatories are not produced in sufficient quantities. This would be enough to trigger such a reaction. Problem: While on 70mg/day of prednisone, a patient is so immune compromised, and has such a decrease in Cortisol caused by the drug, that, should she suddenly stop it, just hitting her thumb with a hammer while hanging a picture, for example, could send her into irreversible shock.

Such patient's normally are weaned from their steroids VERY slowly.... And from 70mg/day of Prednisone she might need the better part of a year to do that.

So what to do? I asked her who her Rheumatologist was, and considering the climate under which Chiropractors at that time practiced; meaning that MD's seemed almost universally to have the attitude that it was their mission to save the world from Chiropractors, I called him, with some trepidation that he wouldn't consider to work with me. But, he was... and it worked great... we agreed that he would monitor her serum Cortisol levels while I recommended a nutritional supplement for her. This was no ordinary supplement, but something known as a Protomorphogen. This was an extract of beef adrenal gland, compounded under the strictest conditions of purity, and with a cold process, which preserved the enzymes and hormones in it.

Bovine, i.e. beef hormones are not active in humans, but the theory was that a human could absorb certain materials from this extract through the mucus lining of the mouth, and the body could cleave off the different part of the molecule which makes it bovine and add, at a great savings in energy, the human part, thus using it as a kind of vitamin, to increase the body's output of normal Cortisol and the other adrenal hormones.

Frankly, I don't know if this theory was ever proven scientifically, but after chewing up some 2-3 bottles at 60 tablets/bottle per day for several months, in conjunction with her Chiropractic adjustments, keeping pressure from her spinal nerves, Cathy was able to safely withdraw from her Prednisone in only 3 months. And, as if by magic, her Lupus stopped progressing!

Remember her 6 month death sentence? One year later she had a child, and managed to survive an additional 18 years. Her family has several times thanked me for the years of life she gained. They cannot be convinced that anything but the intervention of a caring DC made that difference.

Ruptured Cervical Disc

It was the same thing when a young man named Bob Magnone (he has given written permission to discuss his case) came to me after a car accident. He was about 23 at the time. A young man to have suffered what would have become a permanent injury had it not been for Chiropractic.

He presented in my office with extremely severe neck pains, radiating into his shoulders and down his arm. I sent Bob immediately for an MRI, which was in its infancy at that time. My diagnosis of disc injury was more than confirmed, the report showed that his mid-cervical disc was not only herniated, but ruptured.

After discussing the possible effects and risks, I started carefully adjusting his neck initially every day, and then three times a week. In a few weeks, he was out of pain completely.

Still, after that initial diagnosis, his insurance carrier was concerned that he had refused surgery. You see he had first been to an orthopedic surgeon and was told he needed "*immediate surgery*", or he could be "*paralyzed*".

After several months of ongoing care, his carrier insisted on sending him back to their "*consultant*", one Dr. Harvey Nova, the chief of Neuro-Surgery at Englewood Hospital at the time. Remember that Bob was at this time nearly pain-free, almost ready to return to work, and also that Dr. Nova and I knew each other and, I thought had some mutual respect for one another's work.

Regardless, when given the opportunity to recommend that a Chiropractor stop treating, my "*friend*" Harvey, and he was a great Neuro-surgeon, and well respected, still couldn't help taking the opportunity. The AMA would have been proud!

I saw a letter saying that Bob should "*stop receiving forcible manipulation of the neck, as it could be dangerous, and for other reasons, and re-think the recommendation for surgery*". Imagine? He was looking at a nearly asymptomatic individual and recommending that he stop the treatment that clearly had helped him, and go back to have a now obviously unnecessary surgery ???

Lucky for Bob, he trusted my judgment and continued his Chiropractic care. Also, I was lucky, in that I was able to talk to the claims examiner at the carrier, and we agreed that Bob would go back for a second MRI, and if it didn't show significant changes for the better, then I would agree to send him back to a neuro-surgeon.

He went back to have an MRI, and a few days later I got a call from the Radiologist:

Radiologist: Hello, Dr. Press?

Me: Yes

Radiologist: This is Dr. _________, I'm calling about Mr. Magnone

Me.: How can I help you?

Radiologist: Tell me Dr., did Mr. Magnone have surgery on his neck?

Me.: No

Radiologist: How can you be so sure?

Me. Because I have seen him at least three times a week for all this time.

Radiologist: There is NO evidence of any disc injury now!

Me: So much for quackery, huh?

Radiologist: Well, I guess the truth comes in black and white!

He offered to write this up together with me for the medical journals.... Being too busy, I just never found the time to organize this, but with 20/20 hindsight, I really should have done that.

Harvey Lilliard redux

While in Chiropractic college, we are all regaled by the, we assume, apocryphal stories about the "*Founder*", Daniel David Palmer, and his progeny, Bartlett Joshua and grandson David Daniel Palmer, who was living when I graduated from their namesake College. In fact, my class was the last to receive a Diploma from the three famous Doctor Palmers.

According to the legend, the first D.D., who was like many physicians in that era, largely self-taught, became enamored of the vertebral column as the seat of all "*innate intelligence*", and thus the cause of all dis-ease. It wouldn't be until much later that science would play catch-up, and begin to realize that "*innate intelligence*", and homeostatic, self-regulating systems were part and parcel of the same thing. And, that interference with the flow and/or function of the signals through the central nervous and autonomic nervous systems, indeed can be related to the changes in chemistry or other functions, which are as it turns out, the pre-cursors to many organic dysfunctional states.

However, according to the legend, Palmer, while working in Davenport, IA, near where the college still dominates the landscape, was trying to communicate with an African-American custodian there named Harvey Lilliard, who was supposedly "*stone deaf*". Lilliard communicated, somehow that he recalled an incident in which his "*neck went 'pop' and my hearing just stopped*". Palmer examined Lilliard's neck, and snapped a vertebra back into place, and Lilliard could suddenly hear again.

Naturally, after all our studies of neurology and anatomy, etc., we had classes filled with real skeptics about the veracity of this legendary re-discovery of Chiropractic. I too really didn't think much of the story, that is until Mr. B showed up in my office complaining of severe neck pain and radiations into his arm. He was about 78 years old at the time, and was wearing not one but two serious amplifier systems to hear. In fact, he had to have his shirts specially tailored to get them with two breast pockets to hold the aids, which were of necessity too large to be in-ear units.

After a complete exam, and x-rays, and discussing his situation, as is my norm, I was given his ok to commence treatment for his neck pains.

When I adjusted his neck, like Lilliard there was a distinct "*pop*", and he was immediately forced to turn his hearing aids nearly off, due to the volume becoming suddenly too loud. In fact, by the time he left the office that afternoon, he had removed both aids and could hear fine without their help… for a while. After several days, he would find that he began to need the aids and started turning up the volume, until he was at the maximum setting, and then would come back into my office for a "*tune-up*", whence he would leave once again, without the benefit of hearing aids.

This continued nearly until the end of his life, and I think the last time I saw Mr. B was about a month before his passing several years later.

Vision changes

Hearing wasn't the only sense that was changed and improved while patients were treated by my ministrations.

Miss K, came into the office much the same way as Mr. B did, that is, with neck pains and headaches. I immediately noticed that she was wearing coke-bottle thick glasses.

We commenced treatment for her neck pain and it completely disappeared, along with her headaches, but one day she came back for a follow-up visit, and wasn't wearing her usual binoculars. I inquired what had happened, fully prepared to hear that she had undergone some radical new eye surgery. I was truly amazed to hear that she, AND her optometrist both attributed her good fortune to the Chiropractic cervical adjustments she had been receiving. Her vision, had mysteriously and spontaneously returned to near 20/20 !

Zhulin at the Garden

One afternoon, I got a frantic call from Maya Usova. "*Stephen, this is Maya*". "*Yes Maya?*" "*Stephen, come quickly, Sasha has hurt himself*". I ran into the City to look at him. The looks on their faces alone told me a story. Sasha was obviously in pain, and desperate to skate that evening. I examined him and told him, "*Sasha, there's no way you're skating tonite*". He looked really down, and said… "*Do you understand what we'll lose?*"… I said "yes, *Sash, I imagine the appearance fee for this evening's performance*", He said "*yeah $15,000.00 !*"… I asked …"*how many more shows are there in the tour?*"…"*35*"…. I said…"*ok, 35 times $15M, or nothing times 15M... your choice*"… "*??*" Well, I went on… "*if you skate tonite, I predict that they carry you off the ice -on a stretcher to a hospital and you'll have surgery, AND you'll not skate another show this tour.... Or, you can listen too me and finish the tour....*" He said.. "*I think I'll listen to you... but YOU have to tell Tom Collins*"… I said "*ok*". And told Tom.

Their biggest concern was what would happen with Maya? After all, they were already separated and the tour was going on to Orlando, FL the following Friday nite. I just said, "*Maya, you go ahead to Orlando and we'll see if Sasha can meet you there or not*".

Sasha and his girlfriend, now his wife, Tanya came back to my home and we put them up for three days. The next morning I took him for an MRI, and stayed so we could all read it together. There was not one, but two Herniated Discs.

Over the next three days, I innovated a new means of therapy. "*Intensive Chiropractic Therapy, with modalities*". I adjusted him six or seven times a day during this period as well as gave him Ultrasound and Traction… and together we went over his routine, and redesigned a critical lift to take the strain off his low back. It worked! He was back to the tour in Orlando and completed the 35 more shows without incident…. The Athletic Trainer with the Tour was flabbergasted.

It is cases like these, which make all the aggravations of always having to prove one's profession to the World worthwhile.

Chapter 17

A New Life, A New Leaf

**

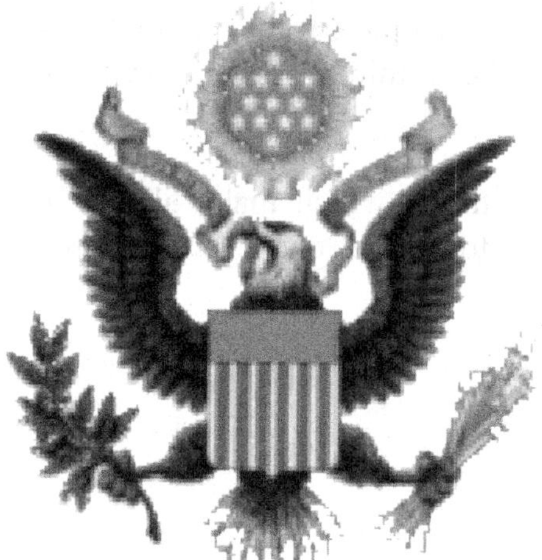

Dad Passes

In February of 2003 I am out to lunch with my friend Dr. Bill Cirino, when my brother calls. He says, "*are you sitting down*?".... I was in my car. My dad had gone out of the house to play golf that morning, and simply dropped his club midway through a basket of balls, and just fell dead on his face. My best friend in the World was gone. My life forever changed. At least he didn't suffer.... only we did. He and mom were together since they were children. That she has adjusted to life without him is yet another evidence of her remarkable personality.

Online Dating

All my woman troubles can be summed up in a short phrase... "*failure to listen to my inner voice*".... Women seem born able to hear and listen to that voice, but guys typically ignore it to their detriment.

When I started to date after leaving Tanya, I realized several facts; one, that I had had my kids and wasn't really interested in starting another family; and, two that I wasn't going to settle for someone I thought I can live with again, but I would wait until I find someone I can't live without.

The Internet, and frankly being able to speak Russian, really revolutionized my dating life. Due to the internet dating services, there were literally hundreds of eligible women interested in dating me at any one time. And, the cutest and brightest of them were all Eastern European. I quickly discovered that this was where my future love life was going to be.

First of all, when I would see a lady of the age and looks I wanted to get to know better, if she was an American gal, about one in ten or fifteen would answer my instant messages. If I saw a Natasha, or Yelena, and started the conversation with *"zdrastvuite, kak delo krasavitsa?"* (Hello, how are you beautiful?) I got about 8 or 9 out of ten answering me.... I quickly found I could be out every night of the week with a different gal..... so, it didn't take a rocket scientist to figure out it was a seller's market. Thus, no longer any reason to "s*ettle*" for less than I really, really wanted. I played the field for almost two years, and then I met Olga.

Olga

I really think that less stable men would have put a bullet through their brains long before I got through this enormous mess. But through it I seem to have gotten. Managed to pay the support, barely, and despite the best efforts of the Family Courts; opened a new office out of financial necessity on Madison Ave, and then, found the love of my life.

My Olga was online... and this time was not in Brooklyn, but here in Jersey, in my own backyard.... And she was gorgeous! And a pediatrician, retired after twenty years in practice in St. Petersburg, Olga was here, happy, and self-assured.... Calm, rational, and emotionally stable, and no huge ego.... A good mom too, she has one son, Alexei studying at Ramapo College. Babies just run towards her.... She's an angel.... The living kind. This reminds of the story about the two guys talking in a bar. One says to the other: "*My wife's an angel*!" The other retorts, "*you're lucky, mine's still living*". We hit it off in every way from the first second together.... Olga and I are compatible in every detail of our lives like I have never felt with anyone before. We just clicked.

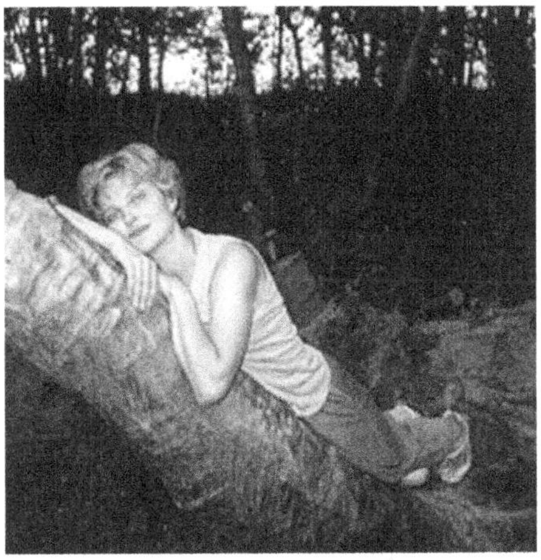

Fig 17 My Olga

I recall a line from the movies….. "*you had me at hello*"…. It's such a joy to come home to someone who really, really loves you…. To your best friend…. To someone who really understands and desires you.

Where is the future taking me? At this writing, I am only 56. There's a lot of time left, I hope…. But I know now that my priorities have changed…. I really want to be home with my Olga. Now, with love in my life too, I have everything anyone could ask for….even the practice is once again growing; and all I have to do is keep her as happy as she keeps me…..

The beginning

INDEX

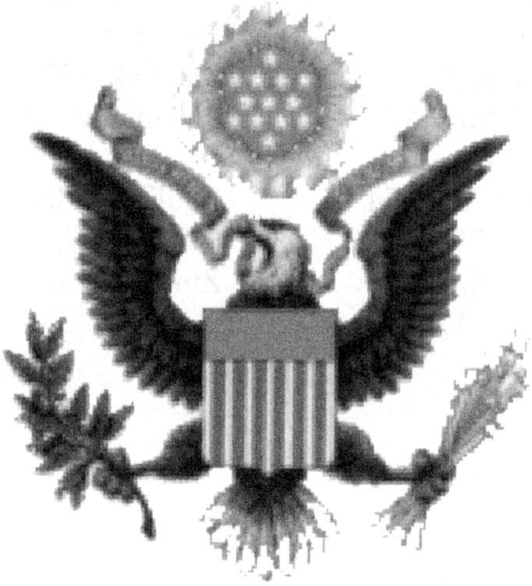

Made in the USA
Monee, IL
08 November 2026

67971944R00129